Best of Small Press Publishers
Minneapolis, Minnesota

*A Candid Approach
to Grief and Death*

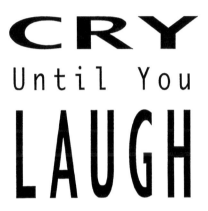

CRY
Until You
LAUGH

RICHARD J. OBERSHAW,
MSW, LICSW

foreword by
Ronald E. Cranford, M.D.

Best of Small Press Publishers
Minneapolis, Minnesota

Best of Small Press Publishers
14550 28th Avenue North
Minneapolis, Minnesota 55447

Best of Small Press Publishers' books are available at special discounts for bulk purchases for sales promotions, premiums, fund-raising, or educational use. For details contact:

Best of Small Press Publishers
14550 28th Avenue North
Minneapolis, Minnesota 55447
1-800-708-0558

Cry Until You Laugh: A Candid
Approach to Grief and Death

ISBN 1-889279-00-5
Library of Congress Catalog Card Number: 96-085913

Publisher's Cataloging in Publication
(Prepared by Quality Books, Inc.)

Obershaw, Richard J.
    Cry Until You Laugh : A Candid Approach to Grief and
    Death / Richard J. Obershaw. — 2nd ed.
    p. cm.
    1. Death—Psychological aspects. 2. Grief. I. Title
BF789.D4O34 1996   155.937
                                      QBI96-40215

Senior Editor: Linda J. Rening, Ph.D
Book & Jacket Design by C H A S
Manufactured in the United States of America

10   9   8   7   6   5   4   3   2   1
First Hard-Cover Edition, January, 1997

dedication

This mixture of ideas, emotions, research and
history called a book is dedicated to the following:
Mr. Ray J. (Penny) Eckstein, Mr. Clarence Novitzke, and
Mr. John Werness, funeral directors that gave me the valuable
opportunity to be close to the bereaved as a funeral director;
Dr. Robert Fulton, Dr. Elisabeth Kübler-Ross, and Mr. Charles Young,
who ignited my desire to better understand and interact with the dying
and the bereaved; my family and friends who encouraged this book; my
professional staff who worked the extra hours during this endeavor;
and, above all, the numerous patients who trusted me and shared their
pain and recovery with me so I might learn to help others
*—*they *are the real experts!*

Special Acknowledgment: William Lamer's *"Sequential Reaction to Loss,"* was reproduced with permission of the author and taken from a lecture given to the Wisconsin Funeral Directors Association, 1966.

contents

preface to the second edition

I wrote the first edition of this book for the grieving people who came to my counseling office and attended my seminars. As a therapist, I had come to realize the tremendous need for a book that was a compassionate, straight-forward companion through the grieving process. So, I wrote that book. Now, after having sold close to 20,000 copies of the first edition, I know that the need for this book extends much farther than the walls of my office and the lecture halls where I speak. Grieving people everywhere need the support this book offers.

Just as the first edition was, this book is written for anyone who has suffered a loss. It will clarify your experiences in the process of grief, and help you to redefine yourself after your loss. This book is also for anyone who is close to someone who is grieving to use as a resource to better understand and support the person who is bereaved. As you will learn, grief is not limited to those who are left after the death of a loved one. Grief is also experienced by people who have been divorced, separated, disabled, or lost their job. Sometimes, even events that we expect to be entirely positive —like the birth of a child or graduating from college— cause grieving because they mean that our identity and way of life have changed dramatically.

The way this book is written meets the needs of people in grief. When we are in pain, we don't want to hear about the theories of pain, or what the experts think of the process of pain, we just want to stop hurting. The same is true for anyone who is grieving. Grieving people don't need theories and research, they need to come to understand themselves and be supported through their pain. So, this book is designed to be easy to read and easy to comprehend. It uses examples, illustrations, humor, and the age old art of storytelling to guide you through your grief.

You will find that this book is candid. It describes in an honest, down-to-earth way the things I have seen, heard, and experienced in my years of work with people who have lost someone or something significant to them. It also offers a practical look at grief and a practical approach to dealing with grief.

I have tried to confront the expectations, myths, attitudes and prejudices about grief that pervade our society. Often, people in grief are hurt again and again by others who are well-intentioned, but who have unrealistic expectations, unhealthy attitudes, and who perpetuate myths about grief and loss which simply are not true.

You may decide to read this book one hour at a time, one minute at a time, or to devour it in one sitting. However you choose to read it,

I hope this book is helpful as you work to process your grief and redefine yourself. Throughout the book, you will find humor is gently inserted to help you laugh a little. This is not to make light of a serious topic, but to help alleviate stress in order to facilitate the learning process. After all, we only laugh at that which is serious.

Those of you who are trying to understand the bereaved will appreciate the stories about other people in grief. They will help you see some of the things people do while grieving, and to be more tolerant of the bereaved. I have learned storytelling is a method which offers a smooth and relaxing way to learn about a bumpy and stressful topic.

Whether you are grieving or you are close to someone else who is grieving, I hope you will come to see grief as a friend and ally that can remind you of your need to change and redefine yourself in every stage of life. If this book guides only one more person in that process, it has been well worth the effort.

—R.J.O.
Burnsville, MN
Summer, 1996

foreword

by

Ronald E. Cranford, M.D.

Combining an enormous amount of clinical experience with a sensitive and common sense approach, Dick Obershaw has given us an extremely helpful, practical book on grief and its many facets. His observations, thoughts, and insightful analysis, coupled with many case histories to illustrate his major points, will be of tremendous value —both to those going through a grieving process and those professionals who deal daily with people who grieve.

After reading this book, no one can doubt the extensive experience Dick has accumulated over the years. Now he shares his thoughts and experiences with us in a highly readable, thought-provoking manner interspersed with his unique humor. There should be more books like this in all areas of health care: clinical professionals shareing their extensive experience so that others, both clients and Health Care professionals, can benefit from these careers.

The book uses concrete examples to help us understand Dick's major themes. Why the JELL-0 brigade should never use paper plates, sunglasses for Hawaii and grieving over the death of a mean husband are just a few of the delightful stories that Dick uses to clarify the myths and realities of grief and mourning. Dick gives us practical, useful insight into the grieving process and the myths of grieving, and compellingly tells us why funerals are so important.

Dick integrates his unique wit and charm into this book, introducing laughter into a deadly serious subject. I strongly urge Health Care professionals dealing with grieving clients to benefit from the wisdom and practical advice of this professional, who has had an extraordinary career in grief counseling.

—Ronald E. Cranford, M.D.

CRY

Until You

LAUGH

CRY Until You LAUGH

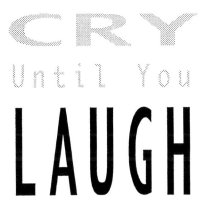

LAUGH

chapter one

We, the Survivors

What is Death? Death as Weird, Unbelievable and in Bad Taste. How Does Our Society View Death? The Future of Death in Our Society. Death as a Force in Our Lives.

At some point in our lives, we will all face death. Whether it be the death of a loved one, the death of an acquaintance, or the death of a hero, death is the *only* thing in life we can count on 100 percent. All of life will eventually end in death, even our own lives. But, until we are dead, we are survivors. And as survivors of death, we will likely experience grief.

To most of us, grief means much pain and heartache, an incredible inconvenience in the least. But each and every day of our lives, we incur loss. And we experience grief for each and every loss we incur. It is after we gain a clearer understanding of grief —after we learn how to work through the grief that results from small losses in our everyday lives— that we begin to grow. We can then begin to gain the strength and knowledge required of us if we are to work through the grief that results from major losses in our lives, losses from death, divorce, or disabilities.

There are some very important questions that, when answered, can give us a more accurate understanding of this thing called "grief." Those questions are: *What is Death? Who is Dying in Society Today?* and *How do We, as a Society, View Death?*

What is Death?
The word —death— has been around for a very long time. Consequently, you would think finding a clear definition of the term would be easy but, it's not as easy as it sounds. To begin, we can turn to the dictionary for a definition.

Richard J. Obershaw, MSW, LISCW

The folks at *Merriam-Webster* tell us, DEATH is "...a permanent cessation of all vital functions." Then they suggest we read on to the definition of brain death. The term BRAIN DEATH came in to being in 1968 and means "...the final cessation of activity in the central nervous system, [especially] as indicated by a flat electroencephalogram (EEG) for a predetermined length of time."

You can imagine how important it is that staff at hospitals and morgues have a precise and accurate answer to the question, when is someone actually dead. A group of lawyers and physicians worked hard to come up with the criteria: a 52-word paragraph that can be summed up in the words: "A FLAT EEG."

A number of years ago, I was privileged to participate in a seminar with life support and trauma unit professionals in a major Midwestern city. Some excellent physicians spoke in the morning, and I was responsible for the afternoon program. One morning speaker presented material regarding the physiology of death. The entire morning, the audience sat around discussing donor organs, transplants, ethics, and the physiology of death.

The speaker began by first asking, "When is a person dead?" Responses from the audience included: when all body functions cease; when there is no response to the environment; and, when the body is pulseless, non-breathing. Then, someone brought up the 52-word sentence, and offered these words to summarize, "Simple, when there are *no brain waves.*"

Cry Until You Laugh

The speaker projected an overhead transparency on a screen at the front of the room. The overhead depicted the printout of an *electroencephalogram,* or "EEG." The EEG was flat, most of the way across the page. But at the far right side of the EEG was a minuscule bulge in the line. The speaker asked us if this EEG signified death. "No, that is not a flat EEG." The speaker declared, "Then please excuse me, I have to leave right away and call my colleagues back in Cleveland to tell them the bowl of JELL-O lives on!"

The speaker had projected an EEG of a bowl of JELL-O. He went on to show that, after all those physicians and all those lawyers spent all that time working on the ultimate definition for death, there is no such thing as a flat EEG. He presented additional evidence; projections of additional EEGs taken in the desert. He had found that even sunspots can cause a less than flat EEG.

Don't we even know when a person is dead? One of my very favorite news articles on this topic came from a Boston newspaper. The headline read: TWO SURVIVE AFTER HOURS OF FROZEN DEATH. The article went on to tell about a man who was found in the hallway of a Boston hotel sleeping off a "significant amount of liquor." When found, the man had no pulse and was, to all appearances, dead. In Winnipeg, Canada, just two weeks before, a 20-year-old female had been found lying in the bitter cold on a city street. She had no heart-beat or respiration, and her pupils were dilated.

The reported wrote, "While it took physicians over 2 1/2

hours to revive the man, and the woman's heart had stopped beating for over 4 hours, both victims are recovering today with little evidence of any side effects."

The reporter went on to explain that as many as seven doctors, ten nurses, and several orderlies worked on the woman for over 3 1/2 hours. They performed external heart massage and manual ventilation and finally, they used a technique known as *peritoneal dialysis* —the injection of a warm solution into the abdominal cavity. The woman regained consciousness and was able to talk and behave just like a person coming out of anesthesia. She recovered with no ill effects other than frostbite. The reporter closed the article with the statement, "These unusual cases are causing authorities to again ponder the exact meaning of death." It's true, as a society, we are deeply confused as to when a person is actually dead.

Recently, I heard a story of a family that went to a funeral home to make burial arrangements for a relative who had died at a local hospital. After the arrangements were made, the funeral director called the hospital to find out if the body could be released. A nurse told him no one by that name had died. The funeral director was persistent, though he imagined the family could have given him the name of the wrong hospital. The nurse explained, "Oh, we have a patient here by that name, but he *isn't* dead yet."

Around that time, the federal trade commission was investigating funeral homes throughout the nation. The funeral director was aware of this investigation, and thought that maybe his establishment was one being investigated. So, the funeral director waited. He waited until he was certain that a friend of his, an administrator at the hospital, would be at the office. Then, he called this friend.

"I might have a big problem here," the funeral director began. He went on to tell about the family who had come into his funeral home to make arrangements for a relative. The family had said that the relative died at this hospital, but a nurse told him, "Nope. No one dead here by that name." The administrator later confirmed that person was there. "But," he added, "he isn't really dead, yet."

The funeral director asked, "What do you mean, not *really* dead yet? The family didn't say this was a pre-arrangement. They said that their husband and father had died."

"Well," the administrator replied, "he's being kept alive on life support. But please don't tell the family."

The funeral director didn't understand why the family shouldn't be told. The administrator explained that the first recipient for the patient's donor organs didn't make it to the hospital, so staff were waiting for a second recipient to be found. The funeral director waited until the next morning and again, called his friend.

"Look, *I need that body,*" he began. "The family is coming

in at noon, and they have no idea..." The administrator apologized, but again explained that the person wasn't really dead, yet. The funeral director called the family to explain why the body of their loved one would not be at the funeral home that day. The family became so upset, they eventually sued the hospital. The suit was, in part, the family's response to their attempts to find answers to the questions: *When do we become bereaved? When do we begin our grief? When do we know that our loved one is dead?*

When is a person dead? becomes an especially pertinent question in this day and age, because there are more and more grandmas and grandpas and husbands and wives and fathers and mothers attached to machines to keep them alive. It is a pertinent question today because in the future, as medical technology advances, we will have the opportunity to live longer and longer lives. And the physical and mental health of the lives we live as survivors are totally dependent upon, and parallel to, our ability to grieve loss due to death.

Who is Dying in Society Today?

Perhaps we can better answer the question, "When is a person dead?" when we come to a clearer understanding of who is actually dying in society today.

We can look for the answer to this question in the evidence: bodies of people who have actually been buried. Usually, when a body has been buried, you can be pretty sure that it was determined that the body was dead. And, one of the best places to look for evidence of dead bodies is in a cemetery.

If you've ever been to a historical cemetery —even some up-to-date city cemeteries— you will find many *infant* graves. Back in the early to mid-1900's, children often died of fatal illnesses for which no cures were known. You can imagine, given the progress of today's advanced medical technology, there would be fewer and fewer children dying. But, if you look at today's research statistics, you will be alarmed. Those statistics would have us believe that an extraordinary percentage of children are dying in our society. When you listen to the news, you hear about children dying on the streets, dying from drug abuse, dying from gang violence and teenage suicide, even dying from murder. We are concerned, and rightfully so, if these statistics are accurate and complete.

But our perception of actual fact has become shaded a bit due to sensationalism. For ages, people have attempted to profit from attending to other people's fears. To argue the points of sensationalism and profiteering in today's news media would take an entire book, and I won't dwell on the topic here. However, I think it is important to note that our perception of what is real —that children make up a large percent of the dying in our society— probably doesn't take into account the whole story, which includes decreased infant mortality rates due to the advancements in our medical abilities. It's not uncommon today to see high survival rates for babies born prematurely. And today, there are fewer stillbirths than ever before in history.

Richard J. Obershaw, MSW, LISCW

I get alarmed when people believe the whole story is told after only a few pertinent facts have been proclaimed, especially when the topic is as fundamental as the topic of death, which affects all of us. Of course, it doesn't matter what the topic is, one can always find statistics to support a unique, albeit mistaken, opinion. And oftentimes, when presented statistics on death today, we are shown only a small, grim segment of a much wider, more compelling horizon. We are misled and unfounded fears are the result.

Imagine looking at the statistics regarding death from automobile accidents in your state. You might see that some percentage of people had been tossed from vehicles, some were slammed against windshields, a few may have been trapped in ensuing fires. And then, way down on one side of the chart, you see that one death was due to "congenital syphilis." That statistic comes from a death certificate in some small county that shows the immediate cause of death in an automobile accident due to congenital syphilis. I have a copy of such a death certificate in my archives, and I've often been tempted to offer it to some theology student doing a masters thesis. My point is, if the desire of the statistician is to suggest that unsafe sexual practices may in some way result with death in an automobile accident, he or she could find the proof.

While statistics would suggest that a major percentage of those dying today are youth, funeral directors —the people who see dead bodies before they are buried— will tell you that no matter what is said, more than 65% of all deaths are elderly; people over the

14

age of 65. When you see the statistics on death to children from gang violence, drug abuse and suicides, don't believe that we live in a society where children have a greater chance of dying than their parents. The facts are: people get old, people get sick; and eventually, *every person* on the face of this earth *will* die. It's always been that way and will always be that way.

Still, the fact that the elderly are dying raises havoc with our society. We've all been reading, listening and watching the news, and everything points to the fact that kids are dying, and we've all become experts on the subject. We sit back in our easy chairs, turn on the tv, and we are instant experts.

If you ever watched the TV series, *The Walton's,* you know it is an excellent show. There we see a family made up of three entire generations, all living under the same roof. Boy, those sure were the good ol' days, weren't they? Kids didn't die back then, they lived to a ripe, old age. Back then, there were few incidents of violent death, suicide or fatal injury involving children.

But today, no child is safe. They are all dying. That's what we might believe. But, that's a lie! In the mid- to late-1800's, there were few, if any, three generation families all alive together under the same roof. It hasn't been until recent history that we've had many cases of multi-generation families.

Today, as always, the elderly make up the largest percentage of people dying in society. And the largest percent of those dying are doing so in institutions, hospitals and hospice centers, not in our homes.

How Does Society View Death?

There are times when what we say —and what we do— are different. Consequently, the mixed messages we send and receive only serve to perpetuate an inaccurate —and unhealthy— understanding of a topic. Without fail, our messages serve only to confuse and obscure what is probably, already, an unclear topic. The topic of death is an example.

Many times, I have been asked to speak to high school students, and it never fails, the dean or administrator introduces me, and the introduction always goes like this: "Today, we are very privileged to have Mr. Obershaw as our guest presenter. He is going to help us learn how to cope when someone we know and love passes away." Then my job is to clear up the mistaken impression that people "pass away." When people die, they are DEAD!

Of course, I have many experiences with mistaken impressions, and those experiences go way back. I grew up in a small town in Wisconsin. In my sophomore year of high school, we had a sex education class. The instructor for the class was a very young, very pretty, first-year teacher. She couldn't have been more than 22-years-old. When she stood up at the front of the room on the first day of sex education class, everyone recognized her as the driver's education instructor. Here, the same teacher who had taught us our behind-the-wheel skills was going teach us about *sex!* You can imagine the giggles from us guys sitting at the back of the room. There we were, imagining that sex had something to do with cars. And the poor instructor stood nervously up at the front of the class and assured us, "Now, there's no reason for any of you to be laughing! Sex is a normal and natural topic." And she was showing us how abnormal and unnatural she felt just teaching the subject!

You'd have to admit, we got two very different messages that morning. The first was that driving and sex somehow went together and to us, that was funny. The second was that sex is a serious subject, that there is no reason to laugh about sex. Well, to us, it was a big joke. Here we were, impressionable, young kids who imagined that we would graduate from that class with our licenses to have sex! Sure, it's not so funny now —especially when you consider that *your* kids could be getting such mixed messages in school today.

We give and we get similar, mixed messages about the topic of death. Go to the nursing colleges who teach specialized care to would-be hospice nurses. Ask the administration what they teach students about grief and bereavement: about *surviving* death. You will find that these schools have *limited* curriculum on this very important topic.

Funeral directors and other grief experts know the funeral is really for the living, for the survivors, not for the dead. And then, during funerals, they hide members of the family off in some secluded room to grieve. Where will the bereaved get support? From each other? Highly unlikely.

Richard J. Obershaw, MSW, LISCW

We've heard members of the clergy tell us that we've got to deal with the reality of death. And then they preach about the dead having to "cut loose from the moorings on the ship of life." Throughout the funeral service, they may not even mention the fact that someone died.

Hospitals pay me well to talk to teach their staff how to help the bereaved, how to deal with death and grieving, and how to communicate with dying patients. And then they hide one of the very best communicators of death —*a dead body.* They even go to the extremes of hiding dead bodies in carts with false bottoms(!). Now that sounds absurd, especially since the majority of deaths in America occur in Health Care institutions. As a society, we are sending mixed messages about death.

There has been more written in the past 15 to 20 years on death, dying, grief and bereavement than in any other time-period we are aware of. And much of what has been written confuses, rather than clarifies. In 20 years, our discussions of death and dying have not changed.

Even in prominent hospice centers and terminal-care facilities, staff *can't* say "dead" and/or "died." They can't communicate, can't keep eye contact, can't talk about their own fears of death with other members of the staff —let alone with patients or survivors.

Death as Weird, Unbelievable and in Bad Taste

I don't doubt many of you have seen the TV series *M*A*S*H*. If, by some slim chance, you never saw an episode, you need to know that about 80% of it is humorous and 20% is serious. And the serious part is super-serious. *M*A*S*H* is a story of a medical unit in Korea during the Korean War. At one point in the series, one of the major characters in the series — Henry Blake, played by McLean Stevenson— was killed.

Mr. Stevenson had decided to take a contract with another TV network to do a different series, so the producers had to write him out of the script. And like most other TV soap operas and serials, when a major character leaves the show, they are usually written out through death. You may recall the character Edith in *All in the Family*. And when the character of Bobby Ewing on *Dallas* talked about leaving the show, he was killed off in a season finale. Of course, when the actor changed his mind, the character's death ended up to be "just a dream..."

What I want you to understand and appreciate is that all of these deaths are just "TV deaths." When Henry Blake was not going to be a part of *M*A*S*H* any longer, and when he was written out of the script through death, it was a fantasy death, and entertainment death. It *wasn't* the *real death* of a real person.

You'd imagine that this character's death should have had little or no effect on us as viewers. After all, don't we know the character is not real? But the death of the character did affect us, and it affected us greatly. As fans of the show, we had invested much of ourselves in the characters on the show. And whenever you invest in something and you lose that thing, you will have to divest yourself of that thing. You will grieve, and you will have to work through that grief.

Right after the episode in which Col. Blake was "killed," a large city newspaper ran a story headlined: VIEWERS BLAST TV DEATH. The article stated, "...Switchboards at CBS glowed an angry red last week when Col. Henry Blake was killed-off during the final moments of the show. A source at the Hollywood studio that produces the show said the reaction to the sad ending was 'tremendous.' The networks across the country were jammed with calls and viewers were reportedly generally upset that Blake had been killed." It went on to say that a Los Angeles TV talk show host threatened, on the air, to "beat up the persons responsible for Blake's demise." One network channel logged more that 40 angry and fiery calls of complaint in just one hour, because of "the weird, unbelievable and bad taste conclusion to what had been an entertaining episode."

If you look at the response to what was only a TV death — *for the purposes of entertainment*— and multiply it by about 10,000, you begin to get an idea of how real death is viewed and responded to in our society today. And in a nutshell, our response is that it is *"weird, unbelievable" and in "bad taste"*; rather than what death really is —normal, natural and highly desirable.

✐

Death as Practical

While much of society would have us view death as weird, unbelievable and in bad taste, there is a large segment that would have us see death from a practical, or more sensible side.

Looking at the practicalities of death should be a healthy start on the journey to a more accurate understanding of death. After all, don't some of us just take things *too* darn seriously in this day and age? Isn't part of the reason we have so many problems in society today because we get "too emotional" over things? If we could *remove* our emotions from this thing called "death," and come to a clearer, more practical understanding of death, we'd be better off as survivors.

Well, let's take a look at the casket. There are a lot of emotional reasons for a casket, but let's disregard those for a moment. Can you imagine any *practical* uses for a casket? One, a casket is stronger than a canvas bag. But a canvas bag is more practical from an *economic* standpoint, as caskets can get pretty expensive. A casket does protect a loved one's body, but that's too emotional. Let's try to keep it practical.

So, a casket has handles, and that's practical. A container with handles are makes for easier handling or carrying. I think that's probably the only practical reason for caskets. Sure, caskets can be locked, but unless you believe the dead need protection for jewelry or other valuables you thought to send along, locks on caskets serve no practical purpose. It could take six or eight people to carry a body from funeral home to hearse to burial site, and caskets with handles are practical.

Now there are those of us who think that's just not practical enough. They will suggest that you can use a casket for, say, a wine rack, or a book shelf, or a cabinet for one's high-tech stereo equipment. Or, put it up on some sawhorses and make a bar out of it. Or, line it as a cedar chest and use it for storage at the end of your bed. Or, just keep it open in the center of your living room as a conversation piece.

Society would have us get very practical about caskets. They would have us make an advance purchase of our casket so we can save the trouble and increased expense we would otherwise incur at some point in the future. As if we'll be there at the time of our death, to worry about such matters.

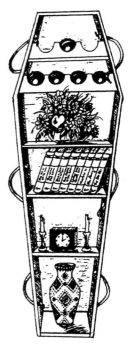

I've spent some time thinking about this, and I honestly don't think that there is anything I could buy today —even a casket— that I could take with me when I die. I believe that dead is DEAD.

The Casket as a Wine Rack.

How about death? How can we make death practical? Some might suggest one way would be to measure the cost of death. We can make death practical, from an economic standpoint, if we measure the cost of a death. For instance, if someone dies in a car accident today, that death costs over *One Million Dollars!* I will itemize this to make it sound more practical. For example: $741,370 in loss of production and consumption in the marketplace; $222,407 in loss to the home, family, and community; $963 for the hospital; $560 for doctors; $455 for the coroner; $3,272 for the funeral; $7,665 for legal expenses; $1,032 for handling insurance claims; $280 for accident investigation; $12,897 in losses to others; $13,965 in car damages; and finally, $280 for delaying traffic.

Okay, that *sounds* practical. But, society would not have us stop there. In many places you can immortalize your loved one, friend or acquaintance by molding their cremated ashes into pottery. Really, they can be *put up in pottery!* You can have flower pots and sculptures made out of your loved ones remains…

Think about it. Practical. A pot keeps on being. It won't take up space —*that's* practical! And, 100 years from now, it will be even more of a treasure as a family heirloom. An artist in a southern state suggests, "It's better to be looking out on the world as a pot, than to be buried under the wet, cold ground." And a reckless young farm kid from Wisconsin suggested to his meticulous mother that his hard-driving father could be molded into the shape of a foot scraper when he died. I'm sure that kid got a weekend tour of the woodshed!

Now, if death is to be practical, we certainly can't have the dead take up space. That's not practical! The United States government doesn't think so either. A few years ago, members of our government became worried about valuable space that is wasted on cemeteries, so they formed a committee to have a hearing. This committee discussed what should be done about wasted space of cemeteries. There was a strong, political faction that suggested cemeteries should be done away with completely because they are just not practical!

Have you ever seen Washington, D.C.? Most of that city is nothing more than one huge cemetery! Everywhere you look, you can see another marker or another monument to some dead person! If we are to do away with space for the dead, we would have to bulldoze that whole city!

Well, I know I'm overreacting a bit so I suggest that we take all of the bodies out of all of our cemeteries and bury those bodies in the medians of our interstate highways. After all, it's federal land. It won't likely be needed for housing developments or shopping malls. We could put flat markers on all of the graves for safety reasons. People comment, "Mr. Obershaw, that's ridiculous! Why, if everyone was buried in the medians of our interstate highways, then everyone alive would be reminded of death every time they drove down the road!"

And I respond, "Yes, sir, they would. And the real reason why people want to do away with cemeteries in the first place has nothing to do with wasted space or practical issues. Research shows that if everyone alive in the United States died today, the bodies could be buried in a space *one-quarter* of the size of our smallest state, Rhode Island!" Those of you who have traveled to North Dakota know that there's enough land out there to bury bodies for hundreds of years to come! (If you're reading this in North Dakota, imagine Iowa...)

No, society does *not* need to move cemeteries for practical reasons. The reason we would like our cemeteries moved is because we *think* death is weird, unbelievable and in bad taste. We don't understand death. We cannot overcome death. And, *we are afraid of death.*

Could you get to heaven faster if you were cremated? That is what some would have you believe. Again, it involves the government. Some time back, our government approved a plan to send cremated human remains into outer space. When the newspaper reported this, the headline read: YOU CAN GO TO HEAVEN WHEN YOU DIE. In smaller printing below, it read: OR AT LEAST TO THE HEAVENS.

The article stated that it would cost each individual about $3,900 for a Florida-based consortium of funeral directors and engineers to orbit a flying mausoleum containing the cremated remains of those individuals by sometime in 1986 or early 1987. It was the first time the transportation department had given approval to a private business to launch a commercial spacecraft.

Richard J. Obershaw, MSW, LISCW

This spacecraft-mausoleum was to carry 10,330 lipstick-sized titanium capsules, each containing the specially reduced ashes for a cremated person. The mausoleum of capsules was to be placed in the nose cone of a privately developed rocket and fired into a circular orbit 1,900 miles above the earth. The orbit was said to be stable enough to keep the remains aloft for "...at least 63 million years, if not for eternity."

In most communities today, it's difficult for cemeteries or funeral homes to obtain zoning permits, so funeral directors in Florida hired engineers and come up with an orbiting mausoleum. No problems then for society; out of sight is out of mind. The orbit was to place this spacecraft in the VanAllen (radiation) belt. There are few inhabitants to worry about so there's no need for hearings and zoning permits. Now, that's practical!

But even more practical was the letter sent to a financial columnist in a large, Midwestern city a few years ago. A reader was considering the practicalities of death when he wrote that his wife was being kept alive by machines in a hospital. He mentioned that the doctors said she could be kept alive for another two months. That would mean that she would not die until the following year. What the writer wondered was, "If I decide to let them continue life-support, and she doesn't die until next year, what difference will that make on my income tax return?... Would I still get to deduct her?" Practical, very practical!

Even a national foundation which fights organ disease would

have us make death more practical. Recently, the foundation ran an ad on the radio, which sounded quite practical.

There you are, driving down the highway and over the radio you hear a voice: "Ladies and gentlemen, did you know that last year, approximately 2,000,000 people died in our United States?" (Music crescendo!)

The voice continues, "2,000,000 people! That means 4,000,000 lungs or kidneys or 2,000,000 hearts or whatever were buried needlessly, and wastefully. Friends, donate your organs. Sign your donor cards today!" (Music, up and out!) Now, how many of those 2,000,000 people who die every year in our country, die with diseased or "dead" kidneys, "dead" lungs or "dead" hearts? The ad is *designed* to appeal to our *practical* side.

Maybe you have seen the TV ad I call the "practically dead ad." The ad cautions viewers— "Don't drink and drive." In the ad, the camera angle is shot from the eye of someone who had been killed because they drank and drove carelessly and recklessly into a fatal accident. The camera angle suggests that the dead drunken driver is looking up to an open grave to his weeping family. A shovel of dirt is thrown in over the camera lens. The ad makes a terrible suggestion; if you drink and drive, you could be killed! But, you won't actually be dead because you will still be able to "look out" of the grave.

Richard J. Obershaw, MSW, LISCW

You can do something foolish and be killed —put in the grave— but you won't be dead. In fact, you will still be around to see your family mourning your death. What does *that* suggest to one who is contemplating suicide? Some people want to commit suicide, in part, to inflict emotional and physical pain on those closest to them. They may also want to relieve some intense pain they feel themselves. And here's an advertisement that suggests, "When you die, you won't actually be D-E-A-D dead." Death will not be as painful or as alone as you might imagine it to be. Plus, all these people who are so close to you will mourn your passing. And as an added bonus, you'll be able to watch!

So finally, through suicide which doesn't really mean Dead dead, the distraught teenager can get his family's attention, the jilted lover can get her revenge, and the confused and forlorn can get some control back in their lives. The message is crazy and absurd. The fact is: when you are dead, you will *not* be in control of your life, you will *not* be able to see out of the grave, and, it won't matter to you whether your family mourns your death or not.

That ad sends a message quite the opposite of its intent. The same case in point is made by a billboard found in many major cities designed to warn children about the dangers of using drugs. The billboard displays all types of illegal drugs and drug paraphernalia with a headline: PUSHERS GET RICH. USERS GET SICK. That billboard says, "Be a pusher, you'll get rich. Be a user, you'll get sick." We get so wrapped up in trying to rationalize the practical side of the issue, we lose sight of the words we say and the message we send.

With all our technological advancements in this, the information age, you might think that our society would, at any moment, begin to spread some truths about death and dying.

That won't happen in a society that continues to refer to the comatose as vegetables. But society would have us believe it is in the best interest of making death practical, that we take the comatose out of the realm of the human, and put them in the place of the vegetative, or vegetable.

But there *is* a method behind society's madness. That method would allow us to continue to do in the future, what we have been doing in the past: harvesting the dead. After all, if we see them as "vegetables," we can harvest them —or at least we can "harvest" the vegetables' organs.

In a large metropolitan newspaper, the headline of a feature article on transplanting organs read: HARVESTING ORGANS. They didn't think you'd read the article with the uncatchy headline: HARVESTING *HUMANS*. That wouldn't be good business! Harvesting vegetables makes more sense, especially when you consider that people today don't die, they "expire" or "parish," or generally just "go bad."

Death as a Mistake

Society would have us believe that death is weird, unbelievable, and in bad taste. When we can't buy that argument, society would have us make death practical. And when these claims don't easily fit our need to deny the reality of death, we try to believe *death is a mistake.*

In a letter to the editor of a newspaper in response to the episode of $M*A*S*H$ I referred to earlier, one viewer wrote she planned to boycott the sponsor's product until the matter was "corrected." We may laugh at that, but it tells me our unreal, untruthful and often perpetuated concept of death, even a "for entertainment only death", is a serious concern.

Recently, a dear friend of mine and I were eating lunch and my friend asked if I had heard the terrible news? Well, there's so much terrible news being reported today, I had to ask, " What news was that?"

"Oh, the news of the 16-year-old boy that died at the medical center," my friend explained. "Why, the parents should sue that hospital." I asked why should the parents sue the hospital? My friend answered, "Well, if not the hospital, then they should at least sue those darn doctors."

I asked, *why* should the parents sue *anyone*, and my friend replied, "Well, the boy went into the hospital yesterday complaining of abdominal pains, and died a few hours later of a ruptured appendix."

Again, I asked why the parents should sue the hospital or the doctors. My friend argued "Come on, Dick, sixteen year-old kids *don't* die of a ruptured appendix. *Somebody must have made a mistake."*

"Nope, no mistake. Kids of all ages die of ruptured appendixes. They do, and he did," was my response.

"Well, then 'he died before his time.'"

"Nope. *It was his time to die, and he died."*

Why would we think a death *must* mean someone make a mistake? Because a *mistake* can be *erased.* Malpractice suites are a kind of eraser for death in our society today. Doctors and hospitals pay billions of dollars a year in malpractice insurance premiums because death is "not supposed to happen." The emergency team didn't respond quickly enough, or the physicians weren't trained correctly, or the hospital didn't have the right equipment to deal with the injury or illness. *Somebody screwed up somewhere* because somebody is dead.

Death *has* to be a mistake. People aren't supposed to die, especially people we love. At least, not until they're of a ripe old age, have had what we suppose to be a full life, and most importantly, don't die until long after we are buried. Maybe, we just do not want to face death because *we are afraid of grief.* Maybe we fear grief because we don't know how to work through grief. Maybe, if we knew how to work through our grief, we could accept the reality of death.

Richard J. Obershaw, MSW, LISCW

Death as Unreal

Certainly, grief can be painful. Oftentimes, *suffering* will accompany grief. Maybe that's why we would rather not accept the fullness and reality of death. But, I think it's simpler than that. I think we know that working through grief means accepting change in our lives, and I *don't* think we like to change. The death of a loved one forces us to change, so, death must be a mistake. If not a mistake, then death must be made practical. If not practical, then death must be weird, unbelievable and in bad taste. If not, then there's only one thing left for us to do: *deny death* completely!

You know of ways we deny death. The most obvious is through using euphemistic terminology —substituting pleasant, agreeable terms for unpleasant or disagreeable ones. You've heard it: people don't die in this day and age, they just seem to "go bad," right? When someone dies, he's said to have "croaked," or "he bought the farm," "deep six'd it," or "bit the dust." Or he's just gone on to "pay the piper," "push[in'] up daisies," "give up the ghost" or "do the lawn-limbo!"

A member of a Midwestern emergency medical team told me that they don't say D.O.A. (Dead On Arrival) anymore; that's too close to reality. They use a new term, T.T.A.D, or *Toe Tagged At the Door.* Down south, I heard it was A.D.D; *All Done Dancing.*

Ever hear of *poetic license?* Once, while listening to a sermon during a funeral, I heard a description of death that was tough for me to swallow. The speaker said the deceased had "cut loose his moorings on the ship of life." Even today, I'm *still* not sure how the deceased actually died...

In big cities, people don't die. They turn into parking meters. You've heard it said; they "expire." Expire, like in "date of expiration?" Like in "he ran out of time, Jack?" What keeps us from saying, "DEAD" and "DIED?" They must be new, four-letter pornographic words, *dead* and *died.*

We have trouble saying dead or died, especially with family members. Sometimes, we think those words are just too much for the survivors to take. We don't want to do anything that might push them over the edge! Believe me, if survivors of death can't hear the words dead and died, they won't hear much of *anything* said to them.

Up north, people don't die. They "pass away" or "pass on." Down south, people just "pass." "You know, old Billy Joe? He pass'd the other day." Down south, people don't pass in or pass up or pass along, they simply pass.

Society would even have us deny death by using euphemistic terms to describe places where we bury dead bodies. These places used to be called *necropolis,* which means *city of the dead.* When somebody sent you to work, "out of the necropolis," you knew where you were headed. Today, you can't be so sure.

First, necropolis was changed to *cemetery.* That's Latin for resting or sleeping place. Society began to have some doubts about the bodies buried in that necropolis; are they really dead or not? They could just be asleep, you know. Better that we call it a cemetery.

It may not be called a cemetery except in horror novels. We call it a memorial park and garden. A *park* and *garden,* where people *recreate* and *things grow.*

Let your fingers do the walking through the yellow pages some day and you might find the Forest Park Cemetery. Sounds nice, doesn't it; a park in the woods. It's probably really peaceful there. You could probably get a lot of rest there, couldn't you? Read down the ad and you'll see that Forest Park is "A Place For Perpetual Care" *as well!* Wow! You can go there as your final resting place and receive perpetual or continuous care. But, when you're dead, are you *really* going to need perpetual care?

If that doesn't suit your fancy, keep looking. How about Pleasant View Memorial Park? Sounds like everybody has a good view in that place. Plus, it's a *memorial* park. Every day someone will commemorate your death. I don't know that's something I'll care much about when I'm dead. Read on, and you learn that Pleasant View provides "pre-need planning." They would suggest that it's in your best interest to plan for the burial of your dead body now before you are dead. That way you will have *fewer worries* when you die...

Trust me, when you are dead, *you won't need* the things

these places can provide. Whether or not your survivors will need what these places provide is something else entirely different. But when *you're* dead, it won't be your problem, much less, something you can do anything about.

Even the people we rely on most to provide us with clear, concise and accurate information at the time of a death would have us believe something other than the truth. If you've ever been to a funeral home, you are an expert on this. Go to a funeral home, and if someone invites you "this way to the slumber room," believe me, you're in the wrong place. There is no body "sleeping" in that room! That is a child-like concept of death. *When someone is dead, that person is* not *sleeping or resting!*

Our denial of death goes beyond the simple use of words and terms to signify death. From layman to professionals, from government to institution, we all play a role in denying death.

The Future of Death in Society

As long as we deny death by continuing to use incorrect synonyms for a word we can't even define, we perpetuate a serious problem. We lead each other down a primrose path of untruth. But then, when you consider that some people suggest no one really has to die at all in this day and age —die as in DEAD dead— you get an accurate picture of where our society is headed in the future.

Have you heard of cryogenic preservation? Cryogenic preservation used to apply to a method used to preserve lab samples. Now, it is used to describe a process of preserving a dead body today, for a cure sometime in the future. And, be sure, the bodies are not preserved in anything resembling a casket. They call it a "forever flask."

Today, people are cryogenically preserved —suspended in a forever flask as liquid nitrogen is vented in and around the body. At some date in the distant future, when the families decide to thaw out the body, they are hoping there will be a cure for the cancer or heart disease or ailment which caused the person to die in the first place.

One woman even had a window installed in her father's forever flask so she could come by on a regular basis to read to him from the daily newspaper! She believes when her father is thawed out, he will be better able to cope because he will have a truer impression of the current state of the world.

Death as a Force in Our Lives

You would think that the answer to the question, "What is death?" would be easier to determine. After all, we are all experts on the subject of death and dying. We may hear that death is weird, unbelievable and in bad taste. We may hear that death can be practical, and if not practical, then denied. One thing we know for certain is that death has tremendous power in our lives. But have you ever stopped to think how that power is manifested?

Cry Until You Laugh

You may not know that life expectancy is 83.2 years for women and 76.4 years for men, if you are born today. Life expectancy statistics are frequently compiled by or for the benefit of insurance companies, and *profit* is the motive behind all of them. Still, they are averages and close enough to serve here as reference.

The reason I suggest that many of you know the power death has over us is because many of you are married. Some of you have families. Do you have any idea why? Did your reason for marrying or having kids have anything to do the reality of death? You are probably thinking it had more to do with *sex* than with *death.* But it is actually related to with death, and one's life expectancy.

Your parents probably got married at a younger age than you did. It's also very likely that your kids will get married at an older age than you. The reason people get married and the reason people have babies —both have a lot to do with death.

When my mother married my father, life expectancy was about 47 years. In that day and age, she, like many of her friends, married young. Many people my mother's age married when they were only early teens because they didn't expect to live much longer than 30 years. When someone, who today is in their 50's or 60's, first got married, they may have been in their late-teens, or early 20's. Life expectancy had increased. Currently, with life expectancy estimated at upper-70's to lower-80's, you see young adults waiting until their late-20's or even *early-30's* to tie the knot! In the future, you may see more people waiting to get married until 50 or 60 years old. If —or when— life expectancy goes up into the 90's, people may decide it's a good idea to study up on this thing called marriage, first. Perhaps people will work at determining what they want in and out of a marriage and will get it right so the divorce rates go down.

Today, most people don't wait until they are older to get married. Most people don't wait to get married because they aren't sure if they'll live to be 50. The thought of death —and maybe, the facts surrounding death— force us to *act,* to *marry,* and to *have children* whether we're ready or not!

Can you imagine: *Death forces us to have children?* Sure, our *fear* of death forces us to have children. And all this time, you thought it was sex, right? But the reality is, for the most part, you don't have to have children. Even considering unplanned pregnancies, you don't have to have children.

Then why do we have children? Because if we do have children, we will never die. *Children imply instant immortality;* you will never die because you will live on through them. And it's likely that you'll spend a good part of your life hoping your children will have children, too.

Remember when you had your first child and you went to show off the kid to your family. You know the scenario: You carried the little bundle into the room and the whole family exclaimed, "Oh yes, *he looks just like you!"* Then your spouse took the child to meet the other side of the family, and everybody exclaims to your spouse, "Oh yes, *he looks just like you!*" Does that give you any idea of which family wants to keep who alive?

A classic example of this happened to me recently when I became an uncle again. When my brother's second child was a two *days* old, my mother entered the door at the other side of the room where my brother was holding his new baby, and shouted, "Oh, it looks just like you, Bruce!" The poor kid was all wrapped up, head to toe, with this little blanket across his face, and my mother thought the child looked "just like Bruce."

We have such a fear of death and dying that we even name our children in ways to keep some person alive. We name our kids "Juniors." We name our kids after grandpas and grandmas. If you are one so named, you understand. Of course, we can always name our child after a saint! That's a great idea, because saints *never* die!

Our understanding of death —or, our misunderstanding of death— forces us to marry. That same misunderstanding forces us to have children. For the most part, death *should* force us to love. But, when we, as a society, start out with an untrue, misleading concept of death, it's no wonder we get other things wrong!

Whether we like the idea or not, death is with us to our end. We can't avoid it, deny it, or redefine it. *Death* will be nothing more, nothing less than what it is: *the end of a physical life, as we know it, on this physical earth, as we understand it.* We know we are not immortal, and because of mortality, death can force us to take a look at life from a very personal perspective.

Even if a funeral director asked the funeral procession to take the quickest and easiest route to the cemetery, I don't think they should! I think that procession should drive right through the middle of town. I think the procession should wave death in front of as many people as possible. Then, that procession might motivate one person to call a loved one and say, "You know, dear, I really love you a lot!"

Or one person might go home that night and sit with his or her partner and ask "Who are we? What's going on with us? What's important in our lives? Why are we doing whatever it is we are doing?"

I like driving through a town where the cemetery is right out on the main road where everybody who drives by has to see it. Maybe when people in that town get to their destination, having driven right by the cemetery, they'll call up their spouse and say, "I love you." Just maybe. Maybe will decide to get out of the crummy job they've hated doing for 20 years and will change their entire lives for the better.

Death should force us to look at ourselves, to examine this thing we call life. Life is a highly desirable thing, but often, people don't see it that way. They only see the pain and suffering because, along with an unreal, mistaken view of death, goes an unreal, mistaken view of life.

We could help ourselves and each other know life. One way to do that is to quit believing or supporting the denial of death and all of the mistaken impressions society has of death. When we begin to appreciate the realities of death we can begin to appreciate the realities and joys of life. And we can begin to share our newfound joys with others.

Death as Desirable

When you think about it, death is highly desirable. How many of us have given 15 minutes of our lives to think about what our lives would be like if we never died? Just think how important death is, how valuable and desirable it is. The only time we generally think about death as being desirable seems to be with suffering, with old age, and with feeling useless.

The words "good-bye" mean: *God be with you.* Today, we've substituted "have a nice day." Because of the law in some states, we say "don't forget your seat belt." I live in such a state, and my wife always tells me that if I died in a car accident and wasn't wearing my seat belt, she'd kill me. Do you ever say good-bye? The other day, when you went off to work in the morning, did you say good-bye to your significant other? Did you actually say "good-bye," or something more like "See you tonight, honey?" Why don't we say "good-bye," good-bye —as if it could be the end of a relationship? First, we don't like to end relationships. Even thinking about that is weird, unbelievable and in bad taste.

Second, we want to believe that we'll see our significant other later, and don't want to imagine any different.

No, we don't end relationships very well. We don't know how to end relationships. Maybe, we are afraid we'll have to start them up all over again, even if it's only at the end of our work-day. I think we need to say "good-bye" more often. And I think we need to *mean* it when we say it. Then, we can begin to work on saying "hello!" *If we work at ending our relationships, we can work at beginning them again.*

I do marriage counseling, and I see numerous problems in relationships as a result of couples never saying "good-bye" to each other. The couples come into my office and tell me, "Dick, we're thinking of getting a divorce. We don't talk anymore. We've both changed. He (or she) is not the same person I married. We've just seemed to 'grow apart.'"

I don't understand how people can "grow apart." These couples live together in the same houses. They eat dinners together at the same tables. They watch some of the same TV shows together, every week. They still have the same kids and sleep in the same bed. How in the world do they grow apart?

I think people grow apart when they don't say "good-bye" to each other every time they part company, even if it's only for a few hours. Then, when they see each other again, they don't say "hello" and begin their relationship all over again.

Cry Until You Laugh

Each and every day, you change. Tonight, you will not be the same person you were this morning. You will have changed, even if in a minuscule way. It's the same with your significant other. If you care about each other, and don't share with each other how you've both changed today, it won't be long before it seems you have grown apart.

Reading *this* book can wreck your relationship with your significant other. If, next week, you respond differently than expected to something because of the information in this book, your significant other will be thinking, "Who *is* this person? We surely seem to be growing apart."

The next time you go to a social function listen to the ways people describe the one you care about. You can tell a lot about your relationship if you find yourself thinking *"Whoa! Has he (or she) ever changed!"*

If you are consistently working at reactivating, rebuilding, and replenishing your primary relationships, you are recognizing the fact that —as real and as inevitable as it is—death *hasn't* happened to you today. You are a *survivor!* Today, you are among the living!

How many times have you heard a survivor mourn, "And I didn't even get to say good-bye!" That sounds the same as, "I never got to say I love you." If you don't end a relationship often and with sincerity, that relationship will always be hanging out there in some incomplete state. If you never say "good-bye," you never really say "hello." Death should force us to do that. Death *should* force us to say "hello," to get to know, once again, the people we love.

You may be aware that between 46% and 50% of all the people who get married today will be divorced within five years. All kinds of people have all kinds of theories behind the statistics, and many theories are valid. People say that the high rate of divorce today is because people are *less religious* than in the past. Or, they will suggest the reason has to do with *social mobility;* people are moving up and out so fast that a close network of supportive friends is never developed. Some will say the high divorce rate is because *women* are out in the *work force* in large numbers, and not around to provide emotional support to the family. There are all kinds of theories, but I think we miss the biggest reason for divorce: Death.

In an age where life expectancy is near the mid-70's, people have many years to ask themselves, "How long will I be able to endure this bad relationship?" When the reality of death comes to us, we are reminded that we may not get out of our relationships alive. It motivates some of us to take a closer look at our relationships, and some of that scrutiny results in divorce.

Death is not weird. Death is not unbelievable or in bad taste. Death will not be made practical. As much as we would like to deny death, death *is* real. It is a part of each and every life on this earth. The fact that each of us will die someday is big news to many people, and I don't understand why. Good news or bad news, it's still reality that people are going to die. *The probability of death is one hundred percent!* In one lifetime, each and every one of us will be dead. D-E-A-D dead —not "expired," not "passed on," not "gone bad" —DEAD.

But, *until* we are dead, *We are Survivors.* And as survivors, death can force us to love; to love life and all that life has to offer. And in that sense, death is highly desirable.

chapter two

The Third World of The Dying

Society's View of The

Third World Worker.

The Care That We Give.

In the past, there were basically two worlds for writers, philosophers and heroes to explore. One was the world of the living, the other, the world of the dead.

The world of the dead, for the most part, was to be found in necropolises —*the cities of the dead.* These necropolises were most often located on the outskirts of a city; because those still in the world of the living were afraid of catching communicable, and often fatal diseases from dead bodies. The living kept this world of the dead way out there, away from water supplies, food markets, dwellings and farms, away from anything that could be infected. When a person died the dead body was ceremoniously carried or moved into this "world of the dead" in a way that everyone could see. The holes for burial were dug just deep enough to bury the body, and a small cross or marker was placed on the grave. Anthropologists have coined the phrase, *the Rite of Incorporation,* to signify this ceremonial ritual.

Throughout history, this rite of incorporation has also been known as the *funeral.* No matter what term is used, this ritual still serves to move bodies from the world of the living to the world of the dead, usually known in modern times as a *cemetery* or a *memorial park.* While the threat of the spread of communicable diseases has diminished, both the ceremony and the cemetery have taken on new and greater importance to those who are still a part of the world of the living. In this day and age, we work diligently to keep the bodies of the dead in the world of the dead. Our fear that the dead might escape their world has led us to build tall rock or spiked fences around cemeteries, and we have installed locking gates. We dig grave holes deeper —up to six-feet or more. Plus we double-lock the dead in caskets and vaults and pile tons of dirt on top after we bury them. As if that were not enough, we put huge stones on top of the graves for extra added security. And when space is at a premium, we might just put the locked casket into a locked vault in a locked mausoleum in a locked cemetery.

Have you ever noticed that —throughout history— the more powerful the individual was in the world of the living, the *bigger* the stone on the grave or the lock on the vault? Even as far back in history as King Tut, all the chambers and mazes of halls and traps of his tomb weren't built just to keep out grave robbers. People were also afraid that the dead body of the King would escape from the tomb to seek revenge and inflict destruction in the world of the living.

For a very long time, one of the most important tasks for the world of the living has been to keep the world of the dead in its place. I don't mean to be sacrilegious, but Christians know how greatly *their* lives have been affected as a result of "one dead person" having escaped the grave...

In this day and age of modern medicine, we don't have to worry about communicable diseases coming from buried bodies of the dead. Contemporary techniques which sanitize and preserve bodies are effective and efficient. But the rite of incorporation is still of great significance now, and the significance that we place on the ceremony and the cemetery has a lot to do with our fears of death.

You have to admit the funeral is of little significance to the dead. If you believe that the dead are not actually *"dead-and-gone,"* but only "passed away," "expired," or gone to some "eternal resting place," then you probably believe the dead actually care about he color of the casket, the music played at funerals, the sincerity, frequency or degree of mourning exhibited by survivors, or the view from their hillside graves. But the real purpose of the rite of incorporation is to attempt to answer the needs and/or fears of the living, not the needs of the dead.

In the past there were only two groups of people who could transcend the two worlds of the dead and the living. One group was the clergy. A priest, minister, or rabbi is still thought to have one foot in the world of the living and one foot in the world of the dead.

The color black has long been associated with death, while white has always associated with life. It is interesting to note that the clergy often wear black uniforms with a little bit of white around the collars —which, symbolically, signifies that they know more about the world of the dead than the world of the living. Because of the clergy's perceived ability to transcend the two worlds, they have almost always been seen as a little weird, somewhat unbelievable and pretty much in bad taste. Remember, that's how we perceive death, and these people "represent" death.

The second group often thought to be able to transcend these two worlds were funeral directors. Initially, all funeral directors had to be members of the clergy. While that is not necessarily true today, funeral directors will usually still wear black, but with more white in their shirts —indicating that they know more about life than the clergy. Still, for the most part, funeral directors are still seen as a little weird, somewhat unbelievable, and pretty much in bad taste.

In small towns across America the clergy and funeral directors are friends. They visit some of the same places, have some of the same hobbies, talk to each other about common subjects, and are generally seen as partners by their community.

Today, there are many individuals who live in both the world of the dead and the world of the living. Many of them are patients in hospitals, nursing homes and hospice centers. Some individuals may be brain dead, some may have dead kidneys, some may have dead lungs. Many of them are being kept alive by life support equipment which keeps their hearts pumping and their lungs breathing. These individuals inhabit the fringes of the world of the dead at the same time they are being kept alive. They comprise *The Third World of the Dying.*

Now because the elderly and the terminally ill still make up the largest percentage of those who die in our society, and because these people are cared for in hospitals, nursing homes, and hospice centers, The Third World of the Dying has grown to include the professionals who work at these facilities. The Third World of the

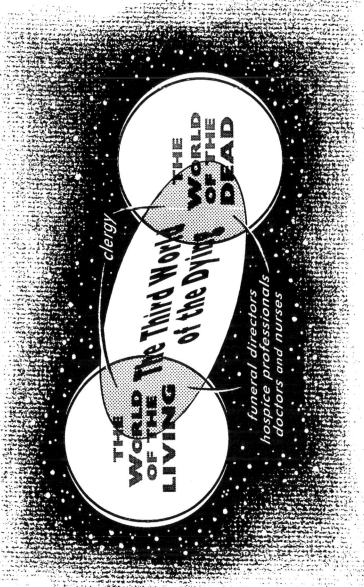

Dying includes critical care nurses, hospice nurses, nursing home staff, doctors, clergy, and funeral directors, plus others who work for or provide care to the elderly or terminally ill.

You might think that many of these professionals would have a true understanding of the reality —and *finality*— of death. While they are very much a part of the world of the living, they work on a daily basis with those who will soon die and become part of the world of the dead. Every day they see the reality of death and the resulting grief. Many professionals appear to be full of life, mentally sound and spiritually alive. At the same time, others appear to be dead to the truth and reality of life, in part, because they have never come to terms with the truth and reality of death. If you work with these professionals, you know that some of these people are emotionally dead. They have no concept of what is going on with the dying, the dead, or the survivors.

Twenty-some years ago we knew little about this third world. What the professionals, patients, and families who made up the third world experienced, believed or felt was largely unknown. That's about the time that a woman by the name of Elisabeth Kübler-Ross wrote a book based on her experiences with death and dying.

Today's graduating nurse is often a nurse who has been death-free. The person didn't attend funerals prior to nursing school, and was seldom around anyone even near death. New nurses may have never even seen a dead body, let alone, touched a dead body. Suddenly, the nurse is told to prepare a body for the morgue. He or she doesn't know how to react to a dead body. Few people, even professionals, can offer any advice.

Elisabeth Kübler-Ross thought that there should be a book of guidance and direction for those who work in the third world so, in the late-60's she wrote *On Death and Dying.* Today, that book continues to sell well because the world of the dying remains unfamiliar and intriguing to the world of the living.

Have you noticed that, traditionally, most nurses wear white, with just a little bit of black? This means that they have lots of training about life, but almost none about death. Consequently, you can imagine how much help they need understanding the world of the dying. Some nurses don't even wear the little bit of black anymore, but to this day, they are thrust into the arena of death and dying. They are constantly called on to make decisions about dying patients' care while, at the same time, having little or no previous experience or education concerning death and dying.

Nurses are the ones most often called upon to decide the "DNR status" of patients (DNR means Do Not Resuscitate). They will say that's incorrect; that *doctors* are the only ones who can make such a decision. But, frankly, that's not true.

Whenever I speak to a group of nurses, I give them the assignment I call "Who gets the heart?" I describe a scenario which includes four patients: a 65-year-old man, a 45-year-old mother with a five-year-old child, a 33-year-old brilliant scientist, and a

25-year-old registered nurse. Each of these patients desperately needs a donor heart to survive, but there is *only* one heart available. I ask them to answer the question— *"Who gets the heart?"*

Invariably, the nurses tell me they don't like "playing God." A majority will tell me that they don't even want to participate in the exercise. Yet, they don't realize they do the same things for real, all the time on the job. Frequently, when a doctor needs to be called in to an emergency, the nurses are the ones who decide the code of the call. Again, they will tell me, "No, Dick. The doctor puts that order on patients' charts, in case the need to resuscitate arises." And I respond, "Wait a minute. How much of the time is the doctor actually there with the patient in such an emergency?"

"Not often."

"Then," I suggest, *"you* are the ones who have to decide if you are going to carry out whatever orders the doctor has written. You decide the code. You decide the DNR status. You make the final decision." The nurses finally have to agree.

The truth is, *they* are the ones who decide.

And doctors often tell me that they don't understand why nurses get so upset on the job. They tell me they —the doctors— are the ones who have to make the difficult decisions of life and death with the seriously ill and the dying. But after I explain the fact, that *nurses* are the ones most often called upon to make the final decision, they tell me they've never given it much thought.

It amazes me the kind of separation and distance one finds in a profession where staff have to work intimately and closely with one another. These people are dealing with life and death and they often aren't even aware of the others' perceptions of reality. And with some, that perception is grossly distorted.

Now, you might imagine that critical-care nurses would have a good idea when a person is dead, especially when they are following a doctor's orders. Research shows when nurses remove the tubes, wires, and monitors from a patient who had been on life support, 80% of those nurses will pull bed rails back up on the dead patient's bed. Why would they pull the rails up? Because some nurses believe the dead patient is only *"a little bit* dead, not DEAD dead." That's the same as believing someone is just "a little bit pregnant."

This professional third world, mostly made up of doctors, nurses, clergy and funeral directors, is expanding to the point where it could potentially include all of us in society. Almost every day, we are called upon to provide care for starving children in another country, to contribute money to research for the prevention of death from some fatal disease, or to protest the untimely deaths of the yet unborn. We are asked to help the dying, support the grieving, protect the unborn —and yet *we can't face* the *reality* of death.

Even a recent best-selling book is designed to help us become more a part of this third world. The topic of the book is suicide. In it, the author tells readers how to successfully commit — or conspire to help commit— a suicide. And all the while, society as a whole has a difficult time accepting the fullness and reality of death and dying.

Recently I was in a morgue in a large mid-western community and ran across an advertisement posted on an employee bulletin board. The ad was promoting a product, the "CCT-100"—or, *Concealed Cadaver Transporter.* I have no idea *how many* CCTs the manufacturer has sold, but I imagine quite a few.

The CCT is a special gurney designed to transport dead bodies. The gurney has a false top that conceals a lower compartment which is properly covered with a sheet. This gurney is wheeled into the room of a patient who has died, and the sheet is removed. The body is placed on the gurney, the sheet replaced over the false top, and the gurney containing the body can be wheeled down the hall — and on and off elevators— with no one suspecting that anyone died.

If an institution doesn't happen to have a CCT-100, they have what I call the "door guard." It's all a part of an institution's "closed door policy." When a patient dies, the funeral director or some staff member from the morgue is called to come and remove the body from the patient's room. When that person arrives, the nurses run down the hallway and close the doors to other patients' rooms. From the end of the hallway, the nurse gives the all clear signal. The funeral director or staff member wheels the body from the room, like a thief in the night, and steals away to the facility's hidden morgue or loading dock.

This is a good example of what I call "team medicine." And I've seen almost *everybody* get into the act. I have seen administrators play the role of hall guard. I have seen clergy shut the doors to other patients' rooms. I have seen doctors and even volunteers give the all clear signal. But it never fails, no matter who's involved in the game, when all the doors are reopened, the patients will almost always ask, *"Who died?"*

Whenever I see this game played, I am amazed. When I ask the staff what they are trying to accomplish. I hear *all* the answers. Most often, I'm told that "hospital or facility policy prevents visitors from seeing dead bodies." Or, "it's bad PR; it's *un-American.*" A few years ago, I read about a lawsuit brought against a major daily newspaper by a hospital. The suit *prevented* the paper from stating the *name* of that hospital in the obituaries. This hospital happened to be one of the best emergency-care facilities in the state, so it received an exceptionally high number of patients in critical-condition. Consequently, a large number died from their injuries, and the hospital became known, not as the "best critical-care facility in the state," but as the *"Hospital of Death."*

Facilities would like to protect visitors who are never supposed to think about death and dying. Or facilities want to protect patients who are never supposed to think about death and dying. Both of those reasons are practical, from an economic standpoint. But, I believe the closed door (of death) policies at hospitals have more to do with the desire to protect hospital staff.

Most hospital administrations are aware that nurses and doctors are very caring, compassionate people. Individuals couldn't be in the profession if they weren't so. They are also very *human.* They build relationships with some, if not all , of the patients they care for. Many times, staff members make sizable investments of themselves in the patients they care for.

They become, in a sense, *extended family* to these patients. This is especially true in critical-care facilities. Patients with terminal illnesses are kept alive longer than ever before, and staff become very emotionally involved with the lives and deaths of these patients. When these patients die —and terminal-illness patients *do* die— the staff will have grief.

The advertisement for the CCT describes the product as a hidden solution to a difficult problem. From all outward appearances, an empty stretcher is being wheeled down the hallway eliminating distasteful experiences for others (staff). The closed door policies in facilities are designed to accomplish the same thing; to eliminate distasteful experiences for staff —the lumps in the throats, the tears in the eyes, the aches in the hearts of the nurses, doctors, clergy and volunteers who have grown to know and love the patients who die. Believe me, those experiences will still be there for these extended family members, regardless of how false the bottom is on the carts, regardless of how long the doors to the rooms are kept shut. You can't shut off the grief that results from loss due to death.

Society's View of the Third World Worker

Many of you reading this book are doctors, oncology nurses, funeral directors, hospice volunteers, or members of the clergy. Maybe, you picked up this book because you or someone you know recently experienced the loss of a loved one due to death. Consequently, many of you are already experts on The Third World of The Dying. You might imagine how society sees you and your relationship with the dead or the terminally ill.

Imagine you are a hospice nurse. All day long, you provide care —emotional and physical— for the terminally ill. If you happen to go to your class reunion, you see once again those friends who haven't heard from you since college. While these friends may have known you were studying to become a registered nurse, that's the *last* they heard. They admired you and your humanitarian goals, but they have no real sense of what you do now for a living.

At the Turn Back the Clock Dance and Reception, you find yourself reminiscing with a couple of old friends. One asks, "Weren't you studying to be a nurse?"

"Yes, and college was grand! That's where I met Bill, my husband," you reply.

"Oh, you're married—? And you probably have a dozen kids of your own," your friends laugh. "So, are you

working as a nurse now?"

You say, "Yes, I'm a shift supervisor at St. Someone-Or-Other's."

"Oh, that's nice! Isn't that just the nice— *Wait a minute!*" they query, "isn't *that* The Nationally Famous Medical Center down south?"

"Why, *yes!*"

They grin with restraint. "Well —isn't that a hospital for children who are *all* dying of cancer?"

And you answer, "Yes...?"

Now, correct me if I'm wrong, but isn't the response you get —or give, depending upon who's talking to whom— something like, "Oh geez. Those *poor kids,* they all die. *Yuck, I'd hate that job!* I couldn't imagine taking care of those kids. *How can you do that?*"

Or if you say, "I work in a nursing home," the response is often, "Yuck! *How can you do that?*"

Or if you say, "I work with people who are dying with AIDS," the response is probably, "Yuck! *How can you do that?*"

Or if you say, "I'm a funeral director," the response will most certainly be, "Yuck! *How can you do that?*"

Cry Until You Laugh

Just tell your friends that you've been doing a lot of reading lately and one of the best books you've come upon is about surviving death and grief. "Yuck! How can you *read* something like that?" is the likely response.

The comments, the questioning looks, the *I-could-never-do-that* are another way of saying, "weird, unbelievable, and in bad taste!" Funeral directors call this response the "hidden-hand syndrome." If you've just made friends with a man who is a funeral director —which is not likely, unless you are one yourself because you are weird, unbelievable and in bad taste— introduce your new friend to others at a social function.

Others will stick out their hands in greeting and ask, "... what is it you do for a living?" When told, they will quickly put their hands behind their backs as if they were just about to touch something weird, unbelievable and in bad taste! Then, they will quietly disappear to the other side of the room because a funeral director *has to be* weird, unbelievable and in bad taste.

Ask yourself if you would get on an elevator for a thirteen floor ride with someone you knew was a funeral director! "Yuck! No way. Don't want to get *too close* to that person!"

A lot of important research has been done on elevators, some quite remarkable. Imagine a pathologist coming to work in the morning in standard business clothes. No one would think twice about getting on an elevator with that person. Put the same person in a smock, and fewer will go along for the ride. Give the doctor a clipboard and an official name tag that says pathologist, and hardly anyone takes the elevator. Smock, clipboard, name tag *and* gurney *with* a covered body—? Forget it! It's a lonely ride on the elevator for that doctor. The more "death-related" the person appears, the less others are willing to relate to him or her.

If you ask your clergy person to come to dinner one evening, and the invitation is declined because the person has to officiate at a funeral, what do you think? If he or she promises to come over right after the funeral, won't you be just a little bit sorry you invited the person over in the first place?

"You'd never catch me doing that for a living!" That's the *weird* part. "How could anyone do that job?" That's the *unbelievable* part. "You brought who to this social function?" That's the *in bad taste* part!

Most of us think there is something weird, unbelievable and distasteful about the people who care for the dead or the dying. But, it's important for us to know how we, as individuals, perceive death and dying, and the people who work with death and dying, in order for us to have a truer understanding of death and this thing called "grief." If we believe that death *is* weird, unbeliev- able and in bad taste, that is *how* we will perceive the dying —*and* anyone who is grieving. As long as we do, we will be unable to provide the care and support the dying —as well as the grieving— need most.

The Care We Give

Much of my work involves listening to and talking with people who work and live in the Third World of the Dying. I have visited with professionals and patients of hospice centers across the country. I have counseled clergy, nurses, family members, and friends who are survivors. And often, I am told how far we fall short in the care we provide the grieving.

Because of our own fears of dying, and our own fears of grieving, we have difficulty distinguishing between the needs of others and the needs of ourselves. My work has led me to assemble a list of needs that I believe many hospice patients have. I wrote this list from a personal standpoint. I tried to put myself in the hospice patient's shoes. It has helped me —as well as others, I hope— to see things from beyond self; from the eyes of one who needs care and support.

HOSPICE: "H" for Hope

As a hospice patient, I would want Hope. I would want a whole lot of Hope. Real, honest and sincere Hope, not unreal, patronizing Hope. As I am faced with my own mortality, Hope is the only thing I know that is eternal. Hope may change, but at the same time, *Hope is Infinite.*

Some years ago, a friend of mine had problems with his throat. He went to a physician, explained that this throat was sore all the time and asked for help. He told the doctor, *"I hope it's nothing serious."* After the examination, the doctor suggested that my friend visit a specialist to have a biopsy taken. My friend said, *"I hope it's not too bad."* After the biopsy, the specialist told my friend he had a malignant tumor on his vocal cords and then scheduled surgery. My friend commented, *"I hope the doctors can get all of the tumor."*

After the operation, the doctor told my friend they could not remove all of the tumor, and more surgery would be necessary. My friend said, *"Wow! I hope I don't lose my voice."* Over the next few weeks, my friend's voice began to fade, to grow hoarse. With what voice he had left, my friend said, *"I hope this won't grow to be too painful."* As the pain increased, my friend was reduced to writing on a scratch pad to communicate with others. One of the first things he wrote was, *"I hope this thing doesn't kill me."* As the cancer spread through his body, the doctors told him he had little chance of survival. He wrote— *"I hope I don't die this year."*

As his strength diminished, my friend worked hard to accomplish the few things he could still do for himself. He began writing fewer messages and developed a kind of sign language to communicate with those who stayed close to him. I remember the gesture he acted out most often; he would wrinkle his eyebrows, smile as best he could, and raise his clenched fist to his chest. That was his sign for Hope.

As my friend lay in his hospital bed, he hoped people wouldn't leave him to die alone. As the frequency of his visitors dropped, my friend hoped that he could die with dignity. When he became confined to his bed, he hoped he was "right" with his God. I sat at my friend's side and watched as his strength diminished, as his hope for a miracle faded. He would look up at me with a feeble smile and squeeze my hand as hard as he could, a sign that he hoped I would not leave his side....

Each and every day, my friend hoped that he could fully live what life he had left. And to the end, my friend's Hope never died. His Hope changed, but it was with him to the very end of his life.

As a hospice patient, I don't want to hear anyone say, "There is *no* hope." I will Hope until the end. And I want others to hope with me, to encourage my hope —even if that hope is, "I hope I can die soon."

HOSPICE: *"H" for Humor*

As a hospice patient, I would want Humor. We all use Humor to ease tension in serious situations. Humor is an important tool which helps us cope. If I had terminal cancer, I wouldn't want others to stop laughing with me. I would want others to joke with me, to tell me funny stories, to talk with me about the crazy things happening in their own lives.

A lot of funny things happen in hospitals. I would want the nurses and doctors to share that humor with me. Funny things happen in churches. I would want the clergy to share that Humor with me. As the time of my death grew closer, I would even want funeral directors to share their Humor with me.

Without Humor, the seriousness of my fateful situation would overwhelm me. And if you can't bring yourself to laugh with me, then at least bring me a book of jokes. Bring me calendars that have a new joke for every day of the week. If I read ahead a few months because I don't know how long I'll live, laugh at those jokes with me, too. Get me a VCR, show me funny movies and laugh with me. Buy me funny get-well cards, and if I can't read them for myself, read them to me and laugh about them with me.

HOSPICE: *"H" for Help*

If I were a hospice patient, I would want Help, a lot of Help. I would want you to *Help Me Die.* Dying would be new to me, something I'd never done before. I would have no idea if I were doing it correctly. I would want you to Help me with my family. I would want more than just the offer of emotional support to my grieving survivors, I would want to *know* that you would Help me to teach my family the things I can't after I'm dead.

HOSPICE: *"H" for Home*

As a hospice patient, I would want to be Home —if at all possible. A large part of my life revolved around my Home. I spent a lot of money providing that Home for myself and my family. I've had some very good times in that Home. Home is a special place to me. I helped design it and worked hard to make it what it is.

I understand there may come a time when I just can't be at my Home. But I would still have that hope. And if that hope changes, I would like to make my room in the hospice or nursing home feel as close to my Home as possible.

HOSPICE: *"O" for Order*

If I were a hospice patient, I would want some Order in what life I had left. I would like to know what to expect, on a daily —*even hourly*— basis. At this enormously disorganized time in my life I would want organization all around me. I would want the phone to be in the same place next to my bed every time I need to use it. I would want my toothbrush and comb where I could reach them and cards and letters close so I could read them. If I have Order around me, I can have some sense of security in the midst of my insecurity.

HOSPICE: "O" for Openness

If I were a hospice patient, I would want Openness. I would need people to be honest and open with me. I would want staff, family, and friends to tell me what's going on with them. If I have your complete and sincere Openness, I will trust you. If you are closed and withdrawn, I will doubt you. I would want to trust that the entire staff —doctors, nurses, and volunteers— had my best interests at heart. I will trust that, if I see Openness.

HOSPICE: "O" for Options

As a hospice patient, I would also want Options. I would want the Option not to be awakened at 5:00 a.m. to be told that breakfast will come at 7:00 a.m. (I can't believe that *has* to be mandatory). I would want the Option to sleep until noon, if I cared to. I would want the Option to have my family sitting on the edge of my bed 24 hours a day, if that's what we need. Don't make visiting hours mandatory, give me some Options. I hope I would at least have the Option to make some choices in what's left of my life.

Richard J. Obershaw, MSW, LISCW

HOSPICE: "S" for Safe

As a hospice patient, I would want to feel Safe. I've *never* died before, so, I would like to have some other people around me going through the same thing as I, so I could check to see if the emotions I feel are normal. Fellowship would help me feel Safe amidst all the mixed up feelings that would certainly be going on inside me.

HOSPICE: "S" for Sex

Yes, even as a hospice patient, I would need Sex. I want you to know that doesn't necessarily mean two hours of passionate love-making. It's much more simple than that. I will need you to touch me, to hold me, to gently squeeze my hand. I will want some tender affection, some intimacy and maybe, some romance.

I may need some time alone with my wife. Again, that doesn't necessarily mean I would need sexual intercourse. It could mean closeness and cuddling and touching and laying together. Don't get the crazy notion that my need for Sex means a need for intercourse. You may remember a time when holding hands was quite sexual. Well, let me be sexual. And let me tell you some jokes I know about Sex. If you can't handle the jokes, send somebody to my room who has a sense of humor.

HOSPICE: "S" for Sharing

If I were a hospice patient, I would want you to Share a part of yourself with me. Sharing is important, because if you know me intimately, I need to know you the same way. You will come to know my private hurts and pains. You will come to learn some of my best

68

kept secrets. And, you will find out some of my darkest fears. I need to know that you are able to give some of the same of you, back to me. If you can't Share such things with me, I will want to know why not. If you are afraid to Share with me, because investing in a relationship with me means you will have to grieve my death, I will Share some things that will help you deal with your grief.

HOSPICE: "S" for Sad

As a hospice patient, I want you to be Sad. I want you to be *really* Sad, too. During the pains for my fatal illness, I will want you to cry. As I'm dying, I will want you to cry. I will want you to tell me you'll miss me after I die. I will want to know, that —after I'm dead and gone— you will mourn the loss of your friend. Your Sadness will make me feel special.

HOSPICE: "S" for Spiritual

If I were a hospice patient, things Spiritual would be very important to me. That doesn't necessarily mean I will need a lot of religious support. That doesn't mean you have to send the chaplain to read to me from the Bible every day. It does mean I will want to talk with you about your philosophies and opinions. I will want to talk to you about life and death and mortality and eternity. To some, Spirituality is music that plays in the background their entire lives. I would like to dance to the sound of that symphony that plays in my life, until the very end.

HOSPICE: "P" for Pain-Free

If I were a hospice patient, I would want to be Pain-Free. I don't think that's a lot to ask for. I'd like to be aware of things going on around me, but as Pain-Free as possible. I will try to remember that I need to experience some pain if I'm going to remain sensitive to others around me. But, in my fatal illness, I will have plenty of emotional pain. And it may be that some physical pain can't be prevented. But I will want pain medication on a predictable, orderly basis. I won't want to have to ask every time I feel the need to be Pain-Free.

HOSPICE: *"P" for Privacy*

As a hospice patient, there might be times when I need Privacy. I might need Privacy for an entire two or three days. Just because I need Privacy doesn't mean I'm depressed; it means I feel the need to be alone.

We've all felt the need to be alone. If you were to come home from work one day to find your family standing in front of your home that just burned to the ground, you would need some support. You would want people to care, to hug, to cry with you. But there will come a time when you say, "I just need to be alone for a while. I need to sort out all of this. I need to sort out all of these feelings I have, and I need to find out who I am now, after this loss."

When I tell you that I need privacy, just shut the door to my room. It doesn't mean I'm going crazy. When I need you again, I'll let you know. I know that's what that little buzzer next to my bed is for. At times I will need Privacy with my God, Privacy with members of my family, maybe even privacy with you. If I need that kind of Privacy, please be able to give me what I need.

Cry Until You Laugh

HOSPICE: "I" for Individual

Even as a hospice patient, I will want to be an Individual with my own identity. I won't want to be just another terminally ill patient in a hospital full of people who are dying. I will still be Dick. I won't want to feel like just another statistic that will live on in some doctor's research paper. I will want to be an Individual —the uniquely human being that I am. I will want to be me for as long as I can be me.

HOSPICE: "I" for Insecure

If I were a hospice patient, I will feel really Insecure at times. I might be afraid of doctors, and you will probably want to make me feel secure. I might be afraid of some forms of treatment, and you will want to give me some sense of security. I will be afraid of dying, and you will try to give me the security of your life. In my illness, your false security *won't* help me much, so at times, just let me be Insecure.

HOSPICE: "I" for Intoxicated

I've thought about this for a long time, and as a hospice patient, I might want to get Intoxicated. I'm not really sure, but one night in my illness, I might just want to get *really* drunk. If I do, I would want you to watch over me so I don't do something crazier than I normally might, and so I don't hurt myself or someone else.

I might want to get Intoxicated, and if you don't give me the liquor I need to get drunk, I'll figure out a way to get it myself. Maybe, I'll call it pain. I know that if I call it pain, I have at least one friend who would smuggle me enough booze to get the whole

71

hospital drunk. I'm not sure, but if I do feel like getting Intoxicated, I would like you to help me.

HOSPICE: *"I" for Interests*

As a hospice patient, I would still like to have my own Interests. Today, I'm Interested in the variety and excitement life has to offer. If I were dying, my Interests may not be as important to me, but that will be my choice. I don't want you to tell me I can't pursue my Interests.

I am interested in photography. If you see me taking pictures in your hospital, I would like you to help me work out any issues that might arise concerning other patients' rights to privacy. I would like you to help me get my photos developed, and maybe, you could help me frame one or two of my pictures to hang in my room. Don't make it difficult for me to pursue my Interests.

HOSPICE: *"I" for Independence*

As a hospice patient, I would like a sense of Independence for as long as possible. I know, sooner or later, I won't be able to do some things for myself. At some point in my illness, I may grow more and more dependent on others. Even if I become dependent upon you, I would like you to give me some Independence. If the time comes for me to get an injection, let me pick which side of my bottom I get that injection in. It may seem like a small thing to ask, but it will give me a sense that I still have some control in what is left of my life. That may be all the control I can handle, but at least I could be sure I'm still alive.

Cry Until You Laugh

HOSPICE: "C" for Communication

If I were a hospice patient, I would want as much Communication as possible. If there are tubes and wires running in and around me, get me whatever I need to Communicate. It may not seem to you that I'd have much of anything important to say, but I guarantee, what I do have to say will mean the world to me.

HOSPICE: "C" for Contact

As a hospice patient, it will be important to me to have Contact. I will want to maintain Contact with the outside world. I will want to know what the real temperature is outside, and about the only way I would be able to get that information is by keeping in contact through you. If I ask, and you tell me it's hot outside, I will want to know *how* hot? I'll want you to tell me if it's *sweaty* hot or *dry* hot or *cool* hot. Even if the outside world is just down the hall at the nurses' station, I want you to take time to keep me in Contact with that world.

I will want a television, and probably, a VCR. When my family sends me a videotape of my son's graduation, I'll want to watch it on my TV. It would be nice if you made me a videotape of your neighborhood cookout or softball game or carnival, or whatever is of interest to you.

And please, don't tell me *that* can't be done. I know a little bit about this information age. I know that every hospital has a VCR and a camcorder. I know it's not that difficult to make a 20-minute videotape of what's going on in the park down the street. I know what life is, and I'll want to keep in Contact with life until the last possible moment.

HOSPICE: *"E" for Excitement*

As a hospice patient, I would also want a little Excitement. I just love to hear what other people are up to. I know hospital staff do whatever they need to do, sometimes, to manipulate their administrations. Those stories are fun and Exciting to me, and I want to hear them all. I want to hear about who's having an affair with whom. I want to know how you feel about your shift-leader. I want to hear about the place you go to worship. I want to hear about your children. And I promise, I won't share your deepest secrets with anyone. I would have nothing to gain if I did. It's just that I won't want to stop feeling Excitement.

HOSPICE: *"E" for Experiences*

If I were a hospice patient, I wouldn't want to stop having Experiences. When a person is dying, it seems that everyone around that person wants to talk in the past. "Do you remember the day..." "Boy, I'll never forget the time..." "I'll never forget, you laughed so hard..."

All that talk about the past is for the survivors. And my survivors will need to talk as they work through the grief that results from my death. But if I'm not dead yet, please don't dwell in the past. Give me some new Experiences everyday. Teach me games I've never played before. Read to me from a book I've never heard of before. Show me pictures of places I've never seen. I want to know about new things. And if you've heard of some new, experimental drugs being used for other patients who have my same illness, I'd be interested in trying them out as a new Experience. Keep the newness and freshness of life alive for me through Experiences.

These are some of the things that I imagine I would want if I were a hospice patient. To me, very much alive and well and still kicking, they don't seem like too much to ask for. To you, if you were caring for me through my terminal illness, it might be tough. It might be tough for you to give so much of yourself if you are in the midst of grieving a loss due to my illness. But I know — because I work with loss and grief everyday— I know that as you work to provide care for me, you are actually helping yourself. When you give of yourself in the interest of others, even in the midst of your grief, you are able to come to terms with the fullness and reality of what it is you have now, *before* it is lost. And, that work will make your grief *easier* to process.

Trust me!

chapter three

We, the Grieving

Bereavement, Grief and Mourning. Experts on Loss and Grief. Grief as Weakness.

Before we take a closer look at how society views grief and the grieving, I'd like to define three key terms often used when talking about death or loss: *bereavement, grief,* and *mourning.* Sometimes we interchange these terms, and to do so — especially in ignorance— only fuels the fire of misconception, and consequently, inhibits the personal growth process that can —and should— take place in the midst of loss.

Bereavement, Grief and Mourning

Bereavement, grief, and mourning are three separate terms that signify three distinct and separate human conditions. Bereavement is the state of being deprived. Grief is the emotion we feel as a result of being bereaved. Mourning is the expression of our grief, or other feelings, that comes from being deprived. Sometimes, we only associate these terms —especially grief and mourning— with loss due to death. But each and every time any one of us is deprived of something, we are bereaved. We will grieve as a result of being deprived, and we will express those feelings, whether we mean to or not, through mourning.

If you've made plans to have lunch with a friend and that friend calls to cancel or postpone your meeting, you are bereaved (deprived). You may *feel* offended; that's grief. When you go out to the parking lot and flatten all of the tires on your friend's car, *that's* mourning!

If you come home to an empty house, but had expected your

spouse and children to be standing at the door to welcome you with open arms, you will be bereaved. You may feel lonely or rejected as a result, that's grief. If you go to the liquor cabinet, pull out the scotch and pour yourself one, that's mourning.

If you turn on TV to watch your favorite prime-time drama, and the program is preempted by a special address from the President, you will be bereaved (and you may be peeved, too). The deprivation —the loss; not getting what you expected— is bereavement. The peeved part —the anger you feel at being deprived— is grief. How you display that anger is mourning.

If you're driving to work, happen to come upon a traffic detour and get angry, you will be grieving. If you then drive that detour at 20 mph over the speed limit because of your anger, you are mourning. And when the police officer pulls you over to issue you a citation, and you suggest that you weren't really speeding, just "naturally processing your grief through mourning," *that's* visions of grandeur!

In the morning, when your alarm clock wakes you up from a restful sleep, you will be bereaved. If you lose your car keys to forgetfulness, if you lose your child to college, or if you lose your job to company reorganization, you will be bereaved.

In each case, you will grieve and you will mourn. The *intensity* of your grief and mourning will depend upon how much of yourself you have invested in what you have lost.

Cry Until You Laugh

Too often, we only associate grief and mourning with *major* painful losses —like death. But, losses that may seem insignificant to others also bring grief and mourning. It is a myth that if you experience what is perceived to be gain by society's standards you will only feel happiness, delight, and joy. If you win the multi-million dollar mega-bucks-bingo-lottery, all of your friends will expect you to be overjoyed. No more worries for you. You'll have financial security for the rest of your life. You can have a new house, new car, and new life-style. Winning the lottery is a big gain for you.

But, could it also be a big loss? If all of a sudden you were given a check for one million dollars, what would you lose? You would lose your privacy. You would lose your old phone number as well, because you'd likely need to get an unlisted number. You might lose some old friends. At least, you would lose the security of knowing who your real friends are. You might lose your home when you might move out of your old bungalow into a new estate. You might lose your present job, your car, your clothes, your kids, your way of life. You could lose everything you have right now.

If you won a lottery every one of your friends would expect you to be elated all the time, but in fact, you might need some intense grief counseling! If so, be sure to call my office. I make special, long-term arrangements for lotto winners!

To assume that *all loss means pain,* and *all gain means happiness* —is an illusion. Such illusions only serve to perpetuate the unfounded, imaginary fears that keep us from accepting the reality of life. But, we already know that because we are *all* "experts" on loss and grief.

Experts On Loss and Grief

Each one of us has gained invaluable knowledge through our personal experiences with loss and grief. We are all experts on the subject.

If you are a New York Yankee fan, chances are, you are an expert on loss and grief. If you've ever been married, whether or not you've been divorced, you are an expert on loss and grief. If you have kids, or if you have changed jobs or careers, if you have moved, if you've lost your wallet, you are an expert on loss and grief.

Just imagine the things you lost when you got married. You lost your freedom. You may have lost money —at least, the choice to spend your money as you could before you were married. Some people have told me they lost their sanity. Some have told me they lost their fantasies, their privacy, and their last names. One lady from Michigan told me she lost her virginity....

The point is, when you get married, you lose your identity — the person you were before you were married. That is not a small loss! Through marriage, much can be gained, but much is lost as well. But, we only seem to see the gain and we expect that everyone involved will celebrate the happy circumstances.

Do you recall your wedding? Maybe you were standing at

the front of the church, in front of God, with most of your friends and relatives present. Perhaps a group of complete strangers (the "other side" of the family who were on the other side of the aisle) were there, too, and in the background, you heard your mom, your Aunt Sue, or your sister crying.

As you stood in the receiving line, the weeping relative walked up, tears still streaming down her face, and offered you a hug. Immediately you consoled, "Oh, don't cry!" And her response was, *"Happy tears!* Yes, these are just happy tears. I'm so happy for you, I could just..." Sob- Sob- Sob.

Happy tears? You married some clown from Embarrass, Minnesota, and your mom, your aunt, or your kid sister were crying *happy* tears?

Chances are, that woman you had once been close to, would rarely see you again —except at holidays or once-a-year family reunions. That woman perceived a tremendous loss, and yet frequently our response to such grief goes something like, "Now, don't cry, mom. You're not losing a daughter, you're gaining a son!"

Many of you are parents. If you are a parent, you are an expert on loss and grief. You know what you lose when you gain a child: sleep, for one. You lose the freedom to come and go as you please (at least for awhile), for another. You lose your relationship with your partner, too. My wife reminded me of that about four or five days after she brought our first child home from the hospital. She asked me, "Why is it, Dick, that when you come home now, you kiss the baby first and not me?"

That gave me something to think about.

When you have children you are apt to lose your privacy. Ever have a three-year-old child open up the bathroom door and yell, "Hi, dad!"? It only happens at the most inconvenient time. And *only* if the bathroom is next to the family room and it just so happens to be the night you're entertaining your new neighbors(!).

When you have a child, you lose and lose and lose. Yes, you experience much gain, too. But, if you imagine that having a child will mean only gain, who are you kidding? We are all experts on this; we know that when we gain a child, we are in for some big losses. It is just never acknowledged.

It begins in the hospital when you, the brand new parent, are standing in front of what I call the "wonder window." The nurse walks up. You point to the little bundle of joy closest to the window and smile. Did you ever hear a nurse say, "You have my deepest sympathy?" Probably not.

Women reading this might remember what happens a couple of days, weeks or months after childbirth. It's that time when the tears start to well-up inside, and the new mother just *can't stop crying.* Her husband comes home, sees the tears and says, "But dear, you *should* be so *happy!*"

So mother tries to straighten herself up. She tries to control the pain, tries to stop all the tears. The next time she visits the gynecologist, she tells her about all these "feelings."

And all too often, her doctor says, "Postpartum Depression!" But this may not be necessarily true. It can be a terribly incorrect diagnosis. Depression is a serious mental illness. Here, a new mother is just beginning to realize all of the losses she has incurred, and those she can expect to ex-perience —she is just coming to understand the drastic changes happening in her life— and the doctor wants to treat her for depression. All this woman is doing is asking herself, "Who am I now?" That is what grief is all about: redefining who you are now, after a loss in your life.

If you graduated from high school you are an expert on loss and grief. The graduation ceremony is, in reality, one big funeral service to ritualize one big loss. Do you remember your graduation?

Think about it. Everyone, family and friends, was gathered together. All of the graduates wore a cap and gown —quite *solemn* clothing. The music was a slow-paced, somber march —a *requiem.* After everyone was seated, some dignitary went up to the front of the room and delivered a sermon. They called it the "commencement address," but it was really a solemn sermon in observance of the grand finale of high school. They just misnamed it.

I know that, because the one word used most often in high school commencement addresses is the same word used most often in funeral services. That word is Hope. At the graduation, it goes something like, "We *hope* you enjoyed your four years here at Tinker-Toy Tech. We *hope* you go on to make your family and friends proud. We *hope* you enjoy success in your chosen career. We *hope* the rest of your life is filled with wonder and joy."

After graduation was the recessional —another solemn march— signifying the end of the ceremony. Then there was a receiving line, and then all of your family and friends waited for you in front of the gymnasium for pictures. You see a lot of receiving lines and gatherings of friends at funerals, too.

At some point, there were handshakes and hugs and gifts were exchanged. If your high school graduation was anything like mine, all the girls cried and all the guys boasted, *"Amen!* Glad to get out of this rotten place." Then, many of the guys went out and drank to medicate their grief.

At graduation, every child loses. They lose the teachers and the friends and enemies they have had for the past four years, all in one big ceremony. Plus, they lose what has been a way of life for the better part of their lives.

My dad —like many dads in those days— had a rule; when you graduated, you moved out of the house. You had to get out in the world, get a job, get a place of your own. Back then many of us graduates lost our homes. Then, we'd lose our parents, too. I wonder where in the world people get the idea that graduation — like marriage, childbirth, and many other gains in life— doesn't include loss? And we're experts on this!

If you wear glasses, you're an expert on loss and grief. I received my first pair of glasses soon after I joined the military. The first three or four days of life in the Armed Services were tough for everybody. I found myself in a strange place, with strange people, doing some pretty strange things. And for three or four days, I got little or no sleep. At the end of those first days, the sergeant took all new recruits in for a medical exam. The exam included an eye test.

After my eye test, I was called up to the front of the line and some eye doctor bellowed, "Okay, Obershaw, here's your prescription for glasses. Next!"

I stopped there in my tracks, turned to the doctor and said, "Whoa, wait a minute! Wait just-a-minute! I don't think I need glasses, sir!"

He said, *"Oh, yeah? Why's that?"*

"Well," I explained, "The reason I can't see your blasted chart way back there is because I haven't had any *sleep* for three days and three nights."

I'll never forget how curtly he replied. "How is it, soldier, you didn't get sleep *only* in your left eye?"

He did have me there! I didn't know what to say. That day, I learned I needed glasses. I had lost a part of my 20/20 vision, if only in one eye. That was a huge loss, a tremendous physical loss, that I did not want to incur in my life.

If you have had any of a number of physical losses in your life —a mastectomy, a hysterectomy, a vasectomy, etc.,— you know about loss and grief. You are an expert on the subject.

If you've had to relocate because of work, you've experienced loss. Not too long ago, a woman came into my office and told me that she was contemplating a divorce. I asked her why she was considering divorce, and she told me that her husband worked for a major corporation. As a part of his job he was required to relocate often. She told me, "I've had to *move* 11 times in 7 years! I will *not* move again. I want a divorce!"

This woman had experienced some major losses in her life due to her husband's job. Every time she got settled in a new community, her husband got promoted, and they moved again. She lost *another* home, *another* set of friends, and her sense of security *over* and *over again.* Those are major losses —and the result is major grief.

If we don't learn to recognize the losses in our lives, learn to identify the feelings that result from those losses, and learn to work through the grief that results, it isn't long before the losses and the grief build up to the point of overwhelming us. When we are overwhelmed, all we know is that we want out. We want to quit. We just want the sadness and hurt to stop.

And, we will do whatever it takes to make the pain stop.

You may be an expert on loss and grief because you have experienced divorce. After years of working with marriage counseling and grief counseling —I don't think I do both of these together by design— I have come to believe that the grief resulting from divorce is often more difficult to resolve than the grief resulting from death. There are a number of reasons why I believe this is true.

First, there are no funerals for "dead" marriages. There is no "rite of incorporation" for the person who used to live in the world of the married, but now must live in the world of the single.

Second, the relationship with one's ex-spouse seldom ever ends —even after the divorce. When a spouse dies, there is some closure to the relationship. But in divorce, you could always run into him or her at the shopping mail, on holiday, or when he or she picks up the kids for the weekend, etc. With divorce, the relationship is oftentimes never over, never finalized.

Third, until recently, there were few support groups for survivors of dead marriages. Today, more and more divorce groups are there to help the divorced. But, sometimes, even these groups don't provide the care and support necessary, because the groups are not prepared to help members work through the *grief* that results from divorce.

It was only ten years ago that I was asked to speak to a church group about the grief that results from divorce. The church officials invited me under the condition that I not use the word "divorce." Can you imagine how difficult that was? I didn't always succeed, of course. Still, I tried to talk about the "death of a dream." Divorce is, in reality, the death of a dream.

And, it can be more difficult to get in touch with the feelings that result from the loss of something *unseen,* than those from something seen, felt, and lived to the fullest.

I'd like to see the formation of support groups for the newly divorced. I think these groups can provide an opportunity for individuals to get in touch with the reality of what has been lost. I think tremendous support and care can be offered in such a group setting. Oftentimes, there is a strong bond within these groups of individuals all experiencing a similar loss. And maybe such groups will someday develop rituals to signify the death of marriages. These rituals could accomplish the same objectives as a funeral.

Recently, a friend of mine, who was in the process of divorce, heard me suggest the idea of having rituals to signify the end of a marriage. He thought that sounded like a good idea, so he scheduled a funeral for his marriage. He imagined it would be quite a party —a wake of sorts.

My friend invited all of his friends to this wake. He invited his former wife and some of her friends. He scheduled the wake for the day after the divorce was final.

On that day, all of the friends gathered at this man's former home. To commemorate the occasion, he set up a Super-8 film projector and showed a movie of his wedding, in *reverse*. A car backed up to the church. He and his wife backed out of the car and walked backwards into the church. All of the rice went back into the hands of the guests. Back, and back, and back the film went...

My friend imagined this would be a humorous touch to what was a serious situation. And when the film began, there were laughs and chuckles in the room. But, as the movie went on, the room grew more and more quiet.

Finally as the film came to the beginning —as the bride walked down the isle backwards and out of the church into the sunlight— the reality of the divorce hit everyone in the room like a bombshell. For each of us that film was like an open casket at a funeral. In spite of my friend's initial motive to add a bit of humor to this serious situation, there was much sadness in the room.

There were tears, a lot of hugs, and many "good-byes." Even though it was not at all what my friend had expected, it ended up being a very healthy experience for us all. Most of the couples that gathered at that wake have maintained relationships with both my friend and his wife which is *not* typical with most divorces. And in these relationships, there are fewer "hidden agendas," fewer games played, fewer feelings hurt. At the wake, all of us got to say good-bye to the couple we had known so long. The couple got to say good-bye to the old way they used to relate to each other. Everyone had an opportunity to *come to terms with the fullness of the emotions* that resulted from the divorce. Those are *essential* parts of working through grief.

We are all experts on loss and grief because we have all had points of bereavement in our lives. As a result we have had feelings. When we expressed those feelings through mourning, too often it was considered by others —and perhaps, by ourselves— as weird, unbelievable and in bad taste.

Too often survivors are denied the opportunity to experience the fullness of their loss. Because of our misconceptions surrounding loss and grief, we try to protect survivors from what we imagine to be unnecessary suffering. Our misguided desires to protect and support do more harm than good.

From my experience as a counselor, I can tell you one way our misguided desires sometimes ruin marriages. This is especially true in cases of stillbirths. When a woman's pregnancy results in a stillborn baby, the first thing many hospitals do is move the mother from the obstetrics ward down to a general ward. Doctors and nurses tell me they do this because all the crying babies in the obstetrics ward only make the mother sad —as if the mother isn't sad in the first place!

Then the doctors, nurses, clergy, and funeral directors approach the father with open arms. They help the father arrange the funeral service, help the father notify immediate family members, and help the father prepare the baby's body for burial. As this is going on, the mother is left back at the hospital.

That is a good start to a ruined marriage. Because, as this is happening, the father is the one who has the opportunity to experience the fullness of the couple's loss. He can better process the grief that results from the loss because he has the support of the doctors, nurses, clergy, funeral directors, and family. Meanwhile, mother lays there, in her hospital bed with empty arms, and a rose from her baby's casket next to her bed.

And, to make matters worse, someone —a doctor, nurse, clergy or family member— visits her and says, "Now, dear. *Don't cry.* Just be glad you're OK. You can *always* have *another* child."

When the mother comes home from the hospital, she will "search" for her child who was stillborn. She will probably live a good part of her life never having processed the grief of her family's loss, in part because we've taken it upon ourselves to deny her an opportunity to experience the fullness of her loss. We can't imagine this mother is emotionally or physically capable of handling the reality of her loss, so we do our best to hide that loss from her.

When I bring this to the attention of hospital staff, they agree more often than not; mothers don't process their grief over a stillbirth as completely as fathers might. But they tell me the reason is because mothers are different. "Dick," they'll say, "you just don't understand. Mother's have a different bond with their babies. Fathers process their grief better because they just aren't so attached to the baby." And, I whole-heartedly disagree. I believe it is because fathers are the ones who get the best opportunity to experience, and process, the fullness of the couple's loss.

Have you ever wondered why hospital staff may not let the mother see and hold the body of her stillborn baby? Because often staff feel it to be weird, unbelievable, and in bad taste. I've been told that mothers don't need to see the body of a stillborn, because mothers already know what babies look like.

Even when a baby is born healthy, everyone tells the parents how *beautiful* their baby is. And that's a lie. A newborn baby is not beautiful. A newborn is a little ball of scrunched up skin with squinty little eyes and clenched fists, covered with blood, and a little cord hangs out of his stomach. No, newborns aren't beautiful; newborns are ugly. It is the *miracle of birth* that is beautiful.

Parents and family and professionals give mothers such beautiful pictures of healthy babies, but when a mother delivers a stillborn, there is only secrecy. The mother is whisked away from all other mothers with healthy babies in the obstetrics ward and told not to worry, that she can always have another child. And as mother lays there alone, she's thinking, "If they won't even let me see my baby, or touch my baby, or love my baby, it must be horrible!"

When a mother is denied the opportunity to see, to hold, and to say good-bye to her stillborn baby, she will live the rest of her life with some terrible illusions about the baby and the stillbirth. She will have been denied the fullness of her loss and the fullness of the support and caring she might have otherwise received. I think we at least have a responsibility to help a mother deal with the reality of her loss, and not hide that loss from her.

Hospitals have the same out of sight, out of mind policies in the case of amputated limbs. If a person has a limb amputated at a hospital, doctors or nurses rarely show the limb to the amputee. The amputee never has an opportunity to come to terms with the fullness of the loss. Of course, we believe that saying good-bye to an amputated limb —having an opportunity to experience the full reality of such a devastating loss— must be weird, unbelievable, and in bad taste. The amputee is left overwhelmed and unable to come to the realization of the fullness of the loss.

A research study determined that hospitals can reduce phantom limb pain by 40% when staff show the amputated limb to the patient and allow the patient to say good-bye to that limb.

Parents who were allowed to say good-bye to their stillborn

babies, and patients who were allowed to say good-bye to their amputated limbs, are able to *process the fullness* of their grief and are better equipped to get on with the rest of life. But it never fails; whenever I suggest that hospitals show amputated limbs to patients and stillborn babies to parents, the staff respond, *"That's just weird, unbelievable, and in bad taste."*

In the case of Sudden Infant Death Syndrome, it's often the mother who gets the attention and support in her grief. Most often the father gets left out. Friends, doctors, and clergy spend time comforting the mother, but dad goes right back to work. We imagine that he doesn't feel the same flood of emotions the mother feels. Again, we think that mothers must need a greater measure of our support and care because mothers have a different, closer bond to children. That's just not true.

I've always wondered why some survivors, depending upon the nature of a loss, are denied every opportunity to experience the fullness of their loss. When we participate in that denial, we paint awful, often overwhelming, and mostly unreal pictures for survivors. The survivors never come to know the truth of their loss. I think we do so because we view death and grief as weird, unbelievable, and in bad taste.

The media greatly influences how we picture death and grief. You can find examples in almost any metropolitan newspaper. Recently, in a large Midwestern city newspaper ran a picture of a father wailing. The father wasn't just crying, he was wailing, his pain and suffering obvious. In the background was a picture of his home burning to the ground. The headline read: EIGHT KILLED IN HOUSE FIRE. Eight other family members had died in that house fire. The paper presented this picture of major loss and major grief in a photo half the size of the entire front page of the paper.

I can recall seeing this photo and thinking how much that picture was going to upset people in the community. I guarantee you, you've seen it, too. Anytime a picture of mourning is presented, the media receive all kinds of letters and phone calls from people who are quite upset. Our society tends to get very upset when grief and mourning are pictured for the world to see. And , sure enough, it was one week later, to the day, that a *letter to the editor* appeared in the paper regarding the photo of the father and his burning house and family.

The writer of the letter asked the paper to review its policies concerning good taste in pictorial reporting. The reader was repulsed by the paper's consistent, cheap sensationalism and suggested she would never buy that particular newspaper again. "Your hideous (weird) front page shocker of [this city's] grieving father has prompted me to write. Why must you feed people such sickness (unbelievable)? Obviously, your paper lacks imagination and must depend on gory pictures or sickening invasions of privacy to make a buck (in bad taste)."

As you might imagine, this wasn't the only reader who wrote to the editor. A majority of the letters from other readers also complained about sensationalism and invasion of privacy.

I've seen pictures like this in a variety of media, and whenever I do, I come to grips with my own mortality. I go to my wife and kids —and I give them a hug. Whenever I see grief and mourning *pictured,* it does something the written word cannot. It forces me to live life more fully.

I think we *need* to see such pictures. I think we need to show the emotions of grieving more openly.

I don't like it when the TV reporter turns the camera on the grieving, jabs a microphone in their face and asks, *"Well, how do you feel about this loss?"* —that's provocation. But, I don't think people should be ashamed of the public display of grief!

People may not like to see pictures like the one I described, because people don't want others to know they are affected by grief. If you view tears as weakness, you will find such pictures disconcerting. Such pictures show the human side of loss and grief in ways the headlines can't. They show the reality of grief, and the fact is, we just don't like to deal with that reality. But, what if such a public display of emotions surrounding a major loss makes other people feel O.K. about displaying their own grief? Maybe then we could look at our own feelings in a closer light....

Some people believe the grieving should have the right to select with whom they want to share their emotions. They believe when the media prints stories and pictures representing grief, reporters are usurping the individual's right to privacy. Many of us have such strong opinions, but few take the time to find out how grieving people feel about the issue. In the case of the man and family in the example I used, I followed up.

I called the newspaper that ran this photo and obtained a copy of the story. From the story I got the name of the family pictured and the city where they lived. From directory assistance, I obtained the family's phone number and called them.

The man in the picture answered the phone. I told him who I was, what I do for a living, and asked if he could help me by answering a couple of questions concerning his loss and the subsequent newspaper story and photo. The man was more than willing to help me.

I asked him how he felt about the national coverage his family received in their time of loss and mourning. I will quote you his answer: *"Thank God for that photographer. Because of that photo, in my deepest hour of sorrow, I received over 3,000 responses from people across the United States. I don't know what I would have done without them."*

The man went on to tell me that many people sent his family scripture verses, and many sent him books about loss and grief. One nurse from Philadelphia even sent him *my* business card. He received letters from people who had experienced similar, massive losses in their lives. He got suggestions on what he should and shouldn't do after such a loss. He again told me, "I don't know what I would have done without them."

The story proves grief is a very private emotion, but mourning makes grief public. If this man had not been a mourner, the media wouldn't have taken his picture. When you mourn, that's public, not private. There was no invasion of this man's privacy.

We all have private thoughts and emotions. As long as we keep those thoughts and emotions private, no one can do anything to us because of them. Thank God for that! But when we make our emotions public, we become responsible for them.

Every time I open my mouth, I become public. This book makes some of my thoughts and ideas about loss and grief public. I need to accept responsibility for my public display, as we all do. The man in the picture decided to make his private emotions public. Maybe he knew he would get comforted. And no doubt, he needed comforting. When the picture appeared on the front page in papers across the country, it told a lot of other people that they needed to comfort him. I think that's very, very important, because that's very, very real.

I believe it's a good idea to invade people's privacy once their grief becomes public through mourning. Just put your arms around the grieving, and they become more public. Touch them and they become more public. Ask them about their loss, and they will become even more public. You aren't invading anyone's privacy, you are allowing someone to be public, and begin to receive the support and comfort they need in order to process their grief.

One of my favorite theories about wailing and moaning is that when we wail and moan, we are actually trying to get the lost person to come back to us; we are trying to get the one person who will comfort us to hear us. If we cry out loudly enough just maybe what we have lost will come back. We all learned that in childhood. As a child, if we cried loudly enough, we at least got some comfort, some needed response.

If you watch people wail and moan at funerals, you will notice that oftentimes, all of a sudden, the wailing and moaning stops. It doesn't taper down gradually; it just stops! The next time you see that happen, look to see who just came in the door.

At one of my lectures, I showed the audience a picture of a man crying in the arms of a priest. I suggested to my audience that it was obvious the man was not calling out for the priest. I did not know that the same priest was in the audience that day. After my lecture, the priest came up to me and said, "You know, Dick, you were right. That man cried and cried until his brother's casket came into the room."

Sometimes survivors will moan and wail until they see the body of the one they've lost. Seeing that body puts closure on the search, and in effect, brings the dead person back.

Whenever I hear people complain about the media's portrayal of mourning, I wonder *why* the complainers don't just turn the page or switch the channel?   When someone says, "Well, last night, I watched four hours of that TV special, *Remembering Viet Nam.* And it was terrible! Just disgusting. There was so much pain. I can't imagine why producers put that garbage on the tube." I ask the person why he or she watched four hours of it.

I think we need to see public portrayals of grief and mourning in order to experience the fullness and reality of the loss. I think we need to see it so we can understand how others feel about it. I believe it helps us to cope, to say, *"We can survive, because we are not alone in our grief."*

In my home state a few years ago, when television stations showed the aftermath of the bombing on the Marine barracks in Beirut, people actually attacked the TV stations. Protesters said the stations "...infringed on the rights" of family members who survived those killed in the attack. Because people were so upset, some of the stations asked the survivors to come into the studio for what they called a Town Meeting. In an open, live forum, survivors talked about their loss and their grief. A number of them said they appreciated the news media and the coverage the media provided. The survivors were thankful that the fullness and reality of the loss was presented. They also were grateful they had a chance to tell their story to the public. The survivors added that if it hadn't been for the media, they would have been denied the support offered by so many people who would just never have understood their grief. What is grief counseling all about? It's about telling the story of a loss. What is a funeral all about? It is about telling the story of a loss. What was the TV coverage all about?

Media coverage of loss and of mourning for all to see, is like a massive obituary. Sure, there are some kooks who come out of the woodwork. Somebody may send a letter full of hate and misdirected anger, but most responses from the public are helpful, supportive, and extremely beneficial to the survivors.

All I ask is that we keep invading the privacy of grief when we see someone mourning. That's difficult for us, because when we do, we often have to experience some deep, dark, painful feelings inside ourselves. Plus, we know that grief is highly contagious. If your friend is crying over the loss of her husband, and you go to comfort her, you can feel grief begin to come over you. As you stand close, as you open your arms to hug, you catch it completely. When we get upset at the media, it's not because the media is invading the privacy of the survivor, but because the media is invading *our* privacy. We do not want to get too close to our own feelings of pain and suffering.

You would have to admit, it was not easy to ignore those pictures of starving kids in Ethiopia when they were paraded across the screen in a two-hour special. My then six-year-old son and I were watching an educational special on TV about starving children.

101

He came and sat close by me. He took my hand and said, "Daddy, don't make me go there." That was pretty smart of him.

When the media invades our privacy while we are sitting in our living rooms with a full stomach, we may be motivated to do something, however small. Hopefully funerals do the same kind of thing to us by invading our privacy. We should run funeral processions right down the main street of town. Invade every on-looker's privacy and they may just go home and give their kids a hug and say, "I really love you!"

A number of years ago, my best friend's wife died of cancer. I was privileged, along with others, to be a casket bearer. If you've ever participated in a funeral, you know how funeral directors often separate the casket bearers from their spouses. This funeral was no different. As casket bearers, we got to sit at the front of the room, our wives sat toward the back. On the way to the cemetery, we all rode in the same car, our wives all went in different cars. At the cemetery, we all stood by each other, our wives stood off in a different place.

Throughout the funeral I didn't get any feedback from my wife. I couldn't check out my feelings or ask her about her feelings. On the way to the funeral reception, I rode with my wife and I got to ask her what she thought of the funeral. My wife said she thought the funeral went really well except for the way the funeral director closed the casket. She was upset that he didn't pull any curtains when he did so. He closed the casket right in front of everybody, and that upset my wife.

Cry Until You Laugh

I looked at my wife and said, "Dear, you've had your own curtains in front of your eyes all of your life. They're called 'eyelids.' Why didn't you pull *those* curtains down?"

She responded, "I don't know. I guess I needed to see what I saw."

When we are confronted with a picture of mourning in the media, or in real life, we can look at the floor and examine someone's dirty shoes. We can file our nails, count the squares in the ceiling, or close our eyes and pray. There are countless things we can do, but we watch with wide-open eyes, and then we get upset. We watch because we know we need to see the reality of death, grief, and mourning.

If you are a survivor of a death, you see the casket at the funeral home, and you come to accept a part of the fullness of your loss. When you see the casket at the church, and you hear the sermon, you come to terms with more of the fullness of the loss. As you participate in the burial ceremony at the cemetery and see the casket lowered into the ground, you come to realize still more emotions associated with your loss. When you consider all of the emotions and all of the opportunities you have to work through those emotions as you come to terms with the fullness and reality of loss, remember —that still may not be enough. You may have to go back to the grave on some anniversary, on Memorial Day, or another holiday to search and find the reality of the loss.

Throughout this whole process of grieving, life goes on. Every day you are confronted with life's realities, life's losses, and you have to work through the grief of little losses. Think how difficult it would be to face life without the support and strength you gain through each of those small experiences.

In my grief therapy practice, survivors talk about the emotions they experience and, often, their ability to accept the fullness of those emotions depends upon whether there was an open or a closed casket during the funeral. I think it is essential to have an open casket whenever physical conditions permit. Some religious groups would take issue with me concerning that suggestion, because to them, viewing the dead body during a funeral is not traditional. However, many of those groups have very strong, established ritual —some span a year of time— to help survivors work through the process of grief.

Grief as a Weakness

While grief is often seen as weird, unbelievable, and in bad taste, I think there is an even more unhealthy view grief and mourning as being a sign of *weakness*. You've heard people say the words, "And when we told her that her husband had died, she just fell apart."

Or, "You know, at the funeral home, she really broke down. And at the cemetery, she just went to pieces."

Or, "I was talking to him about his loss, and be just came unglued."

Cry Until You Laugh

Have you ever heard: "falling apart," "breaking down," "going to pieces," "coming unglued?" All of these sayings suggest that the normal expression of grief, or mourning, is a *weakness.* My car falls apart; people don't fall apart! Have you ever seen anybody actually fall apart or come unglued? At the funeral home, have you ever heard anybody say, "Excuse me, ma'am, you just dropped your arm?"

What concerns me is that much of my personal experience suggests that one of the major fears of the bereaved is that once they start grieving, they will never be able to stop. It will be Humpty Dumpty time. They fear, in essence, falling apart, breaking down, going to pieces. Then, even all the King's horses and all the King's men, all the counselors and therapists, the nurses, clergy, and doctors won't be able to get them back together again. Unless you really see someone drop an arm or see a leg fall off, you should never say those words, because what you do is obstruct the healthy process of mourning.

I can never forget seeing a man who was just told his wife had died. He was walking down a hospital corridor, and just before he entered his wife's room, a well-meaning nurse ran to stop him. As she told him the sad news you could see the grief come over this man. It seemed to start in his eyes, the wide eyes of disbelief. Then his feet began to fidget. His knees began to shake. I could see his stomach quake and his chest begin to heave. He began to move his hand slowly to his eyes. He swallowed hard, his chin started to quiver, and his lips started to strain.

Just as he was reaching for his eyes, the well-meaning nurse said, "Go ahead, sir, it's O.K. to break down." With that, the man dropped his hand, tensed every muscle in his body, and said, "No. No. I'm all right." He remembered the old saying, *get hold of yourself.* He got hold of himself because he felt he was going to fall apart, break down, or go to pieces like the nurse suggested. And he just wasn't sure anyone would be able to "put [him] back together again."

To this day, I don't know if that man ever did cry over the death of his wife. He was stopped from doing so in the hall of the hospital, and many times since he probably reminded himself big boys don't cry. He probably learned that childhood lesson too well. And maybe, for that man, the mourning never did come. And when the mourning never comes, that's the beginning of bigger problems that can continue with us for the rest of our lives.

chapter four

Working Through Grief

Sequential Reaction to Loss. Tasks of Mourning.

If you remember one thing from reading this book, I hope you remember: there are no stages in grief. There are no stages because grief is a process where we work to identify that which was lost, to identify the feelings associated with that loss, and to re-identify who we are now, as a result of that loss.

Have you ever been asked to go for a ride in a friend's canoe? If you have, chances are good you will be asked to ride in the front of the canoe. The person in the back controls the canoe, the person in front is a rock watcher. The one who owns the canoe is there to steer, you are only there to warn your partner if the canoe is about to strike a rock. The owner of the canoe controls the speed at which you move, as well as the direction you float. You just watch the water ahead.

As a canoe rider, you are asked to do little more than watch for hazards. I liken my job as a grief counselor and therapist to that of a canoe rider. I believe that each of us, whenever we are put in a position to offer help and support to a person grieving a loss, is little more than a canoe rider. The grief someone is experiencing is not ours. It is their canoe. We are only along for the ride.

If someone grieving a loss due to divorce says, "I'm going to sell the house tomorrow," that's a rock. If you hear a survivor say, "Gonna take Johnny out of the will. Why, he didn't stay around for more than five days after dad's funeral," that's a rock.

When the recently widowed says, "You know, I just met the nicest man in our grief group. I know I've only been widowed for fourteen days and he's only been widowed for thirteen days, but we're thinking about getting married." That's a boulder!

Our job is to be up there in the front of the canoe. The stream of everyday life will allow our partners in the back to confront everything they will need to confront as they work through their grief. It's their canoe. It's their stream. They will steer, and we only need to point out rocks and boulders and waterfalls.

Our partners may want to paddle upstream for a while, and all we can do is remind them which way the current flows. We may even be asked to paddle a bit, if our partner gets tired. And when the canoe gets swamped, we won't push that canoe to safety; we will pull it to safety. Likewise, we may be called upon to pull our partners out of any messes they've gotten themselves into as they try to deal with grief. There should be a big sign on grief and mourning: NO PUSHING ALLOWED.

When we think of grief in stages, we imagine that we will be able to push survivors through their grief, to what we believe to be a healthier place. It will never happen. Grief is a process, and the illustration on the following page serves to lay out that process.

The illustration depicts what has been called, *The Sequential Reactions To Loss*. Think of it as a map, a guide you can use as you paddle your own canoe of grief, or as you serve as a rock watcher in someone else's canoe.

Again, there are no stages to grief. This illustration, or map, is something you can use as you process grief. It's here to remind you of the many different routes you can take to get from point A to point B.

If you live in New York City, can you get to Jacksonville, Florida by way of Green Bay, Wisconsin? Yes, you can. Or if you live in San Francisco, can you get to Seattle by way of Mexico City? You bet! There are many different ways to get to the same place. You do not always have to go the shortest route. The shortest route might be boring. Maybe it does not look to you like it offers the best scenery. Maybe you would like to take some detours; you may learn a lot by taking those detours. Likewise, the route you take as you work through grief, and the time to take on that route, is up to you. Remember, it's *your* canoe!

As you will note, the illustration looks like a road that goes in a circle then becomes straight. This reminds us that the feelings and behaviors we experience as we work through our grief are tied closely together. On the inner portion of the circle are words that represent feelings we have as the result of a loss. On the outer portion of the circle are behaviors we exhibit as a result of our feelings. You will witness many or all of these in yourself when you grieve, or in others who are grieving. This illustration can help us identify where we are, or where someone we know is, in the process of grief —not so we can push ourselves or others through the process,

Richard J. Obershaw, MSW, LISCW

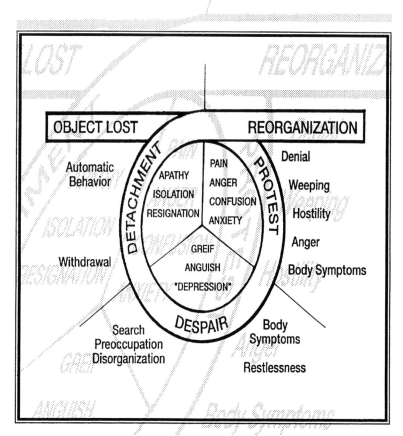

Sequential Reactions to Losses
by DR. WILLIAM LAMERS. M.D.

but just to make us aware of rocks that inhibit personal growth as we work through grief.

Protest

Whenever we lose something, I don't care if it's a job, our car keys, or a loved one, our initial reaction will often be to *protest* the loss.

When a football team loses a down because of an incomplete pass, the team will often protest. You've seen the officials in the booth whose job it is to review plays in instant replay. We do the same reviewing in our own mind whenever we experience a loss. Our initial feeling of needing to protest a loss is a very natural part of the grieving process.

Even though protest is a natural occurrence, it's little more than resistance. Human beings, by nature, are pretty lazy creatures. Research suggests that we use only about 35% to 40% of our full mental and physical capacity. So when confronted with a loss, we protest, because we because we know it will take energy to work through our grief. Do you recall your parents ever having said, *"You spend more energy trying to get out of work than you'd spend if you just did the work."* Well, grief is hard work, and we don't especially want to do it. Loss means *change,* change means *adaptation,* adaptation means *work,* work means *energy.* We don't like to expend energy, so, we protest.

Denial is very much a part of protest. But, have you ever

stopped to think that *denial actually means acceptance?* You cannot deny something without first accepting something. If that confuses you, that's O.K. because confusion is the basis of all learning. And, since the basis of teaching is clarification, I'll clarify—

Some time ago I was driving on the highway and I hit a dog. I was all alone in my car, and as I pulled off to the side of the road, I was saying out loud, "Oh no—! I *couldn't* have hit a dog!"

Sounds a lot like denial, doesn't it? "Oh, no! I *couldn't* have..." But, the last words I said to myself gave it away. I said, *"...hit a dog."* I knew what I knew. I didn't say, "Oh, no I couldn't have hit a giraffe." I knew *my car hit a dog.* I knew which wheel of my car hit the dog. And, I knew it was very likely the dog was dead. I knew what I knew, but that didn't mean I was ready to accept the fullness of what I knew.

A few years ago, I had the privilege to counsel with a elderly woman named Emma, a patient at a Midwestern medical center. Emma was dying of bone cancer, and she wasn't expected to live much longer than a few months. I saw her every couple of weeks to talk about the feelings she was experiencing as she was dying. I recall she used to ask me, *"Dick, I'm a good die'r, aren't I?"*

I had to agree, because she was right. I even told her, "Emma, I wish everyone could be as good a 'die'r' as you are."

Emma was *in touch with her feelings.* She was mentally,

physically, and spiritually *ready* to die, in part, because she worked so hard grieving.

One Saturday morning a nurse from the medical center called me to come talk with Emma. She said, "Dick, you've got to come in and see Emma— I'm afraid she's *gone nuts.*"

"No, *not Emma!*" was my first response. I knew Emma too well to want to believe she was going crazy. I went right to the medical center and the nurse met me on Emma's floor.

"I'm glad you got here so quickly," the nurse greeted me. "Get right in to Emma's room and take a look."

I didn't know what to expect. She had been doing so well; at least, that's what I thought. I hesitated briefly, then went to her room.

There was this dainty 75-pound woman lying in her big white bed, wearing the biggest sunglasses I had ever seen. She had lost a great deal of weight over the past few months, and the big black sunglasses appeared larger than normal against the white sterile sheets. The first thing I imagined was that Emma must have become extremely sensitive to the light —maybe because of the intensive therapy she had been through. Then, I imagined the stark white room must be one big hazy glare to her. Then I imagined all kinds of things about Emma that made no sense whatsoever.

I sat down next to Emma and asked her how she was doing. She was somewhat surprised to see that I had dropped in that Saturday morning, but she was glad to see me. We talked for a few minutes. She shared the events of the past few days, and I tried to figure out if she had actually lost touch with reality.

But Emma didn't seem confused to me. I couldn't imagine what the nurse was talking about. Finally, Emma asked me, "Well, *how do you like them?"*

I said, "What, Emma? How do I like what?"

She declared, "My sunglasses, Dick! Didn't you even notice them?"

I told her, yes, I had noticed her sunglasses. And I asked if her eyes had been hurting her a little bit, with all the bright white in that room, and such. She assured me that her eyes were fine. She had asked the nurse to go to a local drug store to pick up the glasses for her.

"Emma," I asked, "What in the world do you want with sunglasses?"

"Well, Dick" she replied, "I'm going to need them when I go to Hawaii!"

Has there ever been a time in your life when you questioned

your abilities? I had thousands of thoughts running through my head. I could not imagine where I had lost this woman. I had believed she was so "together." She *knew* she was dying. She had worked so hard on her grief. And now, what she said to me sounded like obvious *denial.* I thought I must be in the wrong business! I must have misdiagnosed her somewhere along the line. I just could not remember where it was she slipped by me. All these thoughts were going through my head while Emma and I talked....

Then Emma asked me about Hawaii. I talked at length about beaches, hot sand, and magnificent sunsets. I talked about luaus, fancy pineapple drinks, and big waves. And all the while I talked, I kept thinking— "Dick, where did you *lose* this woman?"

Eventually, feeling somewhat frustrated with myself, I excused myself from the room. I desperately needed a break from all the stormy thoughts in my head. As I walked down the hall, I kept asking myself how I could have allowed this to happen. I began questioning my abilities as a counselor, not just with Emma, but my basic skills from "day one."

As I was gazing out the sixth floor window over a parking lot full of cars moving in and out, I wondered if there weren't probably people down there who would make better counselors than I would. I felt a tap on my shoulder —and turned to see the nurse who had first called me. I'll never forget the biting stare in her eyes as she said, "I was just in Emma's room, and I need to tell you, you didn't do her a whole lot of good!"

Richard J. Obershaw, MSW, LISCW

I was standing there, shaking my head in agreement, ready to apologize for all the years that I had been in this business when the nurse added, "And of all the... Can you imagine— Why, Emma told me she'd *just gotten back* from *Hawaii!"*

And then it hit me! It started in my toes, moved up my legs, through my chest, and into my head. A big smile came to my face. You see, while I was thinking about me, Emma and I were talking about Hawaii. She asked all the questions, I just gave her answers, descriptions and my own story of what little I knew about Hawaii. And, what had looked to me like immense denial on Emma's part was actually great *acceptance.* Emma knew she was dying. She knew the only way she would *ever* be able to visit Hawaii was through someone else: *someone like me!* Imagine the reality of Emma's accepting that simple fact! Emma knew what she knew. Emma knew how one gets to Hawaii when one is dying. I went straight back into Emma's room. I made a date with her for the next evening, and I returned with a slide projector and all the slides of Hawaii I could find. I brought a boom-box to play Hawaiian music and one of those small, drink umbrellas for Emma's ice water. It was a grand evening —Emma got to visit and enjoy just a little bit more of Hawaii.

Three days later, Emma died.

Since that experience I have been very careful to watch for people's denial, because I believe it is an arrow that points to something they have accepted. *And, the more obvious the denial, the more profound the acceptance.*

Cry Until You Laugh

When we attempt to offer support and care to someone who is experiencing grief, we need to deal with what has been accepted. We need to forget about what is being denied. Denial, in its beginning, at its infancy, is therapeutic. It is only one brief stopover on the rocky road through grief.

Denial is one of the very first behaviors we exhibit to protest a loss we incur in our lives. If you had to tell me that someone significantly close to me just died, my first response would likely be, "No! No! He *couldn't* have died!" My hands would go up over my eyes, —I know that if I looked in your face, I would see your message was real. Maybe I could not handle any more reality right then. My next words would probably be, "Tell me you're wrong, you've *got to be mistaken!*" I would even solicit your help in my denial because I might have trouble accepting the reality of my loss.

We need denial. Denial is a kind of buffer zone, if you will; a place for us to stop so we can take in the reality of the information we know to be true. Denial of any loss, even loss due to death, isn't all bad because it is our way of preparing ourselves to accept the fullness of our loss and the feelings that come with it.

Some years ago, a woman came to a funeral home where I consulted. I happened to be there in the lobby dressed in suit and tie. She walked right up and asked me if I was a funeral director. I told her that I was —I was a licensed funeral director in Wisconsin— and she asked me to come out to her car for a moment. I couldn't imagine what this woman wanted. As I walked closer to her car, I looked up and down the street, wondering if, maybe, I was on *Candid Camera.*

The woman opened the back door of her car, and there lay a beautiful brown and white collie. The woman looked up to me and asked, "Is my dog dead?"

I reached in the car, briefly examined the dog, and told her that as far as I could tell, yes, the dog was dead. I thought that perhaps the woman wanted a child's casket or something else she could bury her dog in, but she only said— "Thanks. I just wanted to know if he was *really dead."* The woman had just come from her veterinarian —who told her that her dog was dead— but that wasn't good enough for her. She said that she needed to come and see a "Death Man."

There are levels of denial we can look for as we try to provide support and care for the survivors of a major loss. One sign to watch for is denial that a loss has taken place. For example, there are survivors who have kept the body of a loved one in their home, not telling anybody about it. These people will pour lime over the body —a crude sort of mummification process— and lay out the person's clothes every day. They will do the laundry and cook meals for the person as if that person were still alive. Of course, there are subtler ways to deny the loss of a loved one. A survivor might keep the bedroom just the way the loved one liked it, with the same pictures on the wall, the same sheets on the bed, the same clothes in the closet.

Denial is also evident when one denies —or "distances"— the full meaning of the loss. For example, a survivor may suggest, "We weren't that close anyway." Or, "Well, I kind of expected this death; it's no big deal."

Some survivors will do away with everything that reminds them of the dead person, like taking down every picture of him or her. A married person might selectively forget— "Oh, Niagara Falls? I forgot we went there on our honeymoon! Now, how do you suppose I could have forgotten that? Well, I'll be darned."

Some people will deny the irreversibility of death. At times, that kind of denial takes the form of a spiritual practice or belief. "He's not really dead; he's just in that great workshop in the sky." Sometimes, denial might involve the occult or seances in an attempt to keep in touch with the dead.

Again, I don't know that there is anything we can do to help the grieving move out of their denial. All we can do is point out the rocks that are obvious to us. Whether or not they move their canoe away from a particular rock is their choice.

Another behavior we exhibit in our grief is weeping. Weeping can be a very beneficial outlet for pain and anger.

Researchers have conducted extensive studies on tears.

What they have found is that the tears we shed from emotional pain *are different* from the tears we shed in physical pain.

Briefly, what researchers do is ask people to sit and watch sad movies —real tear-jerkers, like *Brian's Song* (1970). They collect the tears and conduct a chemical analysis of them. The researchers also expose these same people to eye-irritating chemicals similar to the chemicals in onions that might cause tears, and then analyze those tears. The two collections of tears contain different hormones.

Anger and hostility are also manifestations of protest. When anything happens that we cannot, or do not want to accept, we get mad. And, we blame. When someone dies, we hear, *"Damn doctors! If they really knew what they were doing, my mother [or my wife or my kid, etc.] would be alive today!"*

Or we hear, "Damn God! Pastor, tell me about 'your' God. I want to know *why* my loved one is dead. He didn't drink. He didn't smoke. He never chased women. He's dead —and *that man* down the street does all those terrible things, and *he's* still alive! Tell me if that's fair. *Tell me how God could think that's fair."*

Or, "Those damn paramedics. They're *never fast enough.* If they'd just been here a few minutes sooner," or "Damn the funeral director. If he'd never suggested that we *'view* the body,' I wouldn't be so sad. He only wanted to make a buck off my grief anyway!"

We even get angry *at* the dead —really angry sometimes.

But, it's not O.K. to be angry at dead people, so we don't often mention it. Ever hear from a widow who is angry at her dead husband? Widows often feel they have been deserted, and that makes them really angry. Sometimes that anger is veiled, at times it's more obvious. You might hear a widow say, "When George left me, ..." as if George had some choice in the matter.

Recently a widow was talking to me about the death of her husband. I told her that I thought she sounded really angry. "No I'm *not* angry," she snarled.

I told her that it was O.K. to be angry; it was just a rock I was pointing out. But, she couldn't see it. Two sentences later, this woman said, "... And do you know how hard it is to get kids to shovel snow? 95 inches of snow this year, and I can't get the kids to shovel the walks! 95 inches of snow and William *is not here* to shovel the darn walks!" No, she was not just a little angry with her husband for dying, she was really angry at him for dying.

Nurses are, in reality, extended family members of their patients, and when one of their patients dies, they often get really angry, too. A nurse may say, "Sure, I knew he was dying. But *why did he have to die on my shift?"*

It's the same as saying, "How could he do this to me?" It's like there has been a direct, personal attack; and for nurses, it *always* seems to happen at 10 minutes to three —just before their shift ends.

Anger directed at oneself, anger directed at others, anger directed at the dead. But anger doesn't always show itself easily. Sometimes the dog just gets kicked. Sometimes we quit eating foods that are healthy for us, if not all food. We start to have terrible headaches, dizziness, and upset stomachs, diarrhea, back pain, neck pain, menstrual problems, forgetfulness, and insomnia. All these are symptoms of anger without an outlet, anger directed at one's self.

I think women get a constant message from society that says, "It's not O.K. to be angry." That is one of the reasons why women have a higher incidence of going to therapists for depression. It's O.K. for women to be depressed, but not angry. Many women are actually incorrectly diagnosed and treated for depression, because it just isn't O.K. for them to be angry. So, lots of women try hard to be nice when they are angry. But we know, it is most difficult to be nice when we are angry.

When I speak in front of a large group, I like to play a game with my audience. I ask for a volunteer to come to the front of the room, and we play a game of charades. I whisper a word in the volunteer's ear that describes an emotion. The volunteer's job is to act out the word to the best of his or her ability. The audience shouts out what emotion they believe I suggested.

The first word I whisper is ANGER. The volunteer will make all kinds of angry faces: tense brows, frowns, teeth clenched. The volunteer will angrily fold her arms close to her chest and stomp her feet. She will stomp and stomp and stomp until someone in the audience yells, *"Anger!"* That never takes too long; most of my audiences are pretty sharp!

The second word I whisper is FRUSTRATION. The volunteer will make all kinds of sad faces: furrowed brows, frowns, an open mouth. The volunteer will sadly fold her arms close to her chest and take one pace backwards. She will walk backwards: one — two — three steps. No one has fallen off the back of my stage yet, before that happens, someone in the audience will usually yell out, *"Frustration!"*

The third word I whisper is LOVE. Quickly, the volunteer will grab me, hug me, and sometimes give me a kiss on the cheek. I really enjoy being on the receiving end of that word. The audience quickly shouts, *"Love!"* at this charade.

Then I whisper the last word in the volunteer's ear, and step away. The volunteer will stand there with an empty look on her face. In all of the years I have spoken to groups and played this game of charades, not one volunteer has come up with any actions to demonstrate the last word. I assure the volunteer that she is not alone in her bewilderment, that no one ever gets that word. Then, I thank the volunteer, the audience applauds, and I suggest that I will try to demonstrate the word.

I begin by striking my forehead with my clenched fist. Silence in the audience. So I bite my hand. More silence. Then, I kick myself in the rear end, bite my hand, and strike my forehead with my fist, all at the same time (not an easy task, I assure you). Finally, one person in the audience will mumble, *"guilt?"*

GUILT! I hate to use that word, and I seldom ever use it. But, it's the word I was looking for from my audience. Guilt is nothing more than anger directed at self.

But again, you know that. We all know about anger directed at self. We've seen it in others, and we've exhibited it ourselves. And whenever we lose something, we tend to get really angry at ourselves—

"Dumb me! If only I would have taken away his keys, he never would have been driving that car!"

"Dumb me! I should have told him to quit smoking 20 years ago!"

"Dumb me! I could have walked away from that argument, but I had to get right in the thick of it!"

"If only... I should have... I could have... "

And we don't stop with words, do we? We beat ourselves up, physically and emotionally, to neutralize the pain we feel.

You may not have experienced it firsthand, but you know that physical pain neutralizes emotional pain. Actually, physical pain neutralizes physical pain, too. When you wake up in the middle of the night and have to go to the bathroom, you move quietly not wanting to wake your significant other. You don't turn on the light, you just step softly along the side of the bed. And just as you come around the corner of the bed, you drive that little toe of yours right into the edge of the footboard. You have got some serious pain going on in that little piggy, and what do you do? You bite your hand and quietly yell, "Arr*rggghh*h!" Pain neutralizes pain.

Have you ever watched a person take a sliver out of his finger? He will bite his lip, squint his eyes, and gasp to neutralize the expected pain. Have you ever watched a nurse give someone an injection? She will tense up, bite her lip, and squint as she drives that needle into her patient's arm. Pain neutralizes pain.

Whenever we have terrible emotional pain we have a tendency to inflict physical pain on ourselves. When someone loses his job, he will not eat (or, he may *over*-eat). When a parent gets upset with her kids, she might get terrible headaches. Many of us get stomach upsets and back pains when we are experiencing emotional pain.

Some time ago a woman came into my office in great emotional pain. She had all kinds of physical symptoms headaches, back pain, tension-all because she was in terrible emotional pain. She was in so much emotional pain that she said to me, "Dick, I'd pay you anything if you could help me get rid of all this emotional pain. I'm just overwhelmed with pain. It's wrecking my relationships, my job, my whole life!" I asked her how much she would be willing to pay me, if I could help her get rid of her emotional pain. She said, "Well,

I know you can't. But, if you could, I would pay you *anything!"*

I claimed, "No, I *can* help you get rid of your emotional pain! And I'll guarantee it! Now, how much will you pay me?"

She replied, "Oh, Dick. If you could, I'd pay you *whatever* amount of money you wanted!"

I asked this woman how much money she had in her checking account. She told me she had about $2,000 to her name. I told her that would be close enough. For $2,000, I could guarantee that she would leave my office that day with no emotional pain!

With a questioning look she got out her checkbook and began writing out a check for $2,000. I let her write out the amount, the date, to whom, and as she began to sign the check, I told her to stop. I told her to tear up the check. Sure, I could help her get rid of her emotional pain, but I told her that my method wouldn't be ethical....

She sat there shaking her head in "I-knew-you-couldn't do-it" fashion —ripping up her check. I explained, "I could help you get rid of all of your emotional pain, I guarantee it, but it would not be ethical. All I would have to do would be to come over to you and stomp down on your left foot until every bone in that foot was broken. And as the paramedics were carrying you out of my office, I guarantee, you would not be feeling any emotional pain!" The woman glared at me a moment. Then, with wide eyes, she said— *"Kitchen cupboard doors!"*

Cry Until You Laugh

I did not know what she was talking about, so she explained. She told me that, periodically, over the past four months, she would open up a cupboard door in her kitchen, turn to get something out of the fridge or off the counter, and each time she turned back— *whack!* She'd bang her head on the door. She exclaimed, "You know Dick, those were the moments and hours that I can't recall having any emotional pain!"

Often, people in the midst of grief are very accident prone. They may sprain their ankles, wrench their wrists, cut their fingers on cans, or slam their hands in car doors. I am constantly amazed at the number of people who come into my office for grief counseling with fingers bandaged! And as they keep coming back for their next appointments, I can just about tell where they are in working through their grief by the numbers of new cuts and bruises and bandages on their bodies.

✎

Suicide is often one way to give yourself massive physical pain to end some massive emotional pain. Pain neutralizes pain. It always has and always will. I believe that some people see me, a counselor, as one who inflicts emotional pain. People come into my office with some amount of emotional pain, and I challenge them to get in touch with the fullness of that pain-a necessary step if one is ever going to work through whatever is causing them pain in the first place. Then, I charge them for the work I do. My patients may feel some financial pain when they leave my office, but I am O.K. with that, because I know pain neutralizes pain.

Plus, I open doors for my patients. When our session is over I open the office door and let my patient go out ahead of me. All counselors do that, and you think it is just because counselors are polite. They may be polite, but they are also watching their backsides! We know that sometimes when people feel pain, they direct it at others in hopes of minimizing the pain.

You may have seen people give more money than they can afford to their church following the death of a loved one. I know one woman whose three children were all killed in one automobile accident, and she gave $20,000 to her church. In reality this woman was frightened that God was sending her a terrible message through the deaths of her children. It was not my job —especially as a counselor— to tell her she was wrong. My job was only to point out the fact that I saw a huge rock in the way of her processing her grief.

Through counseling this woman and I talked about her pain. We also talked about the money she gave to her church and the reasons behind that giving. She eventually came to understand the reason she gave so much had nothing to do with some perceived, terrible message from God. If it did, this woman would have to grieve the loss of her faith as well, because her faith suggested that God would not send such a terrible message. She came to understand that she gave so much money in order to feel great, financial pain. That was her way of dealing with the emotional pain.

Through counseling she grew to feel better about herself and her relationship with God. And, she eventually worked through the grief she felt over the loss of her children.

When we feel emotional pain, the physical pain we inflict upon ourselves is often exhibited in physiological symptoms. You may have heard of ulcerative colitis —an inflammation of the colon. Ulcerative colitis is a physiological complaint that is often the result of loss and unresolved grief. Research began in the early 1940's and continued today suggests that a high percentage of the people who develop ulcerative colitis do so in close relationship to the loss of a significant person in their lives.

Osteoarthritis —the degeneration of cartilage and bone joints— is also often correlated with unresolved grief and stress.

Recently, two psychotherapists have suggested that cancer may be associated with unresolved grief. These two therapists interviewed women who had recently had pap smears. When a pap smear test is inconclusive, the therapists asked the woman to come back in for another test. The therapists interview the woman at that time, questioning her as to the types of losses she has experienced in a three month to three year period prior to the test. The interview is designed to assess where these women are in their grieving processes.

The therapists measure the responses to the interview questions in an attempt to pre-diagnose the results of the women's second pap smears. In 77% of the cases, they have correctly pre-diagnosed cancer in the women by looking at their grief responses.

Despair

Too often, despair, as it is associated with grief, is misdi-agnosed as depression. Despair occurs when one loses hope or confidence in a situation. It is a psychological response to an emotion, one often associated with loss and bereavement.

Depression is a psychoneurotic or psychotic disorder marked by sadness, inactivity, difficulty in thinking and concentration, a significant increase or decrease in appetite and time spent sleeping, feelings of dejection and hopelessness, and sometimes, by suicidal tendencies. Depression often needs to be treated with psychotherapy and/or drug therapy; despair (grief) does not. We need to be really careful when someone says to us, "Oh, I'm *so depressed!*" If that someone is truly depressed, they need professional help. If that someone is only in despair (grief), don't perpetuate their misconception and misdiagnosis; just point out where you may see a rock.

Most of the time it's fairly easy to tell the difference between despair (grief) and depression. Despair (grief) is a kind of emotional see-saw; up and down, up and down. One minute, the bereaved is up; the next minute, he or she is down.

But it isn't long and that person is back up again. Then it's not long and that person is down. You've heard it: "Oh, I'm so depressed, I can't stand it. But, Jim and I are going out tonight, and maybe *that* will make me feel better. But, we're going to that same restaurant where Jack and I used to go, and now, Jack's passed away. But, Jim's a nice man, and he has a lot of money. But oh, I feel so down. Maybe things will start looking up someday..."

Depression is kind of an emotional submarine: a constant down. When a person is depressed, little or nothing will get them up. Often, the depressed person is heard to say, "So what?...Who cares?...Life's just not worth living....I can't sleep — I can't eat — Who could eat at a time like this?...Nobody loves me....Guess I'll just go out and—"

We also see what appears to be disorganized behavior in the bereaved. But, while they appear to be very disorganized, they are really very organized. The problem is, the bereaved are often only organized towards one thing: getting back what he or she has lost. The jilted lover comments, "I just can't seem to get her out of my mind. Everything I do or everything I see reminds me of her."

The widow may say, "Ah! A paper cup! I remember when Joe drank out of a paper cup just like that one." Or, you will hear, "Oh, look at that light in the ceiling. I can remember when grandpa had a light in the ceiling just like that one."

He or she seems very disorganized, but is actually organized towards one thing. Everything reminds the survivor of the person he or she lost. Of course, most of us are experts on this, because at some point in our teenage years, we lost a boyfriend or girlfriend.

I will never forget the first time I was "dumped." I became, for all appearances, very disorganized. But my mind was very organized toward one thing: getting her back! My school work suffered, because I only thought about her. I started seeing less of my friends, because I spent most of my free time thinking about her. I began to come home late, past my curfew, because I just had to drive by her house 30 or 40 times every night. Every song I heard on the radio just happened to be "our song." All of my energy was focused on one thing —getting back what I had lost.

When you hear survivors of a loss say, "I just can't seem to get him or her out of my mind," you know survivors cannot get him or her out of their minds because they don't want to. If you have ever experienced a major loss in your life, like the loss of a loved one to death, you know the fear of having to give up and grieve for those little things that remind you of what you have lost.

After a major loss in our lives we do not want to experience more grief than necessary. When we lose someone physically, we do not want to have to lose that person emotionally, too. No, working through grief is not fun, so everything serves to remind us of what we have lost, and our hopes are that we will never have to let go and get busy with the work of grieving.

But people close to us care about us. They will tell us to "just keep busy!" Have you ever heard that? When someone says, "I just can't get him out of my mind," we hear someone else say "Oh, just keep busy!" Keeping busy does not help, does it? No, in fact it does more harm than good.

Let me give you an example of why keeping busy doesn't work. I want you to keep reading for awhile. Do not put this book down right now even though someone just ran into your parked car out front.

Now, I know you didn't hear the crash, because you were so engrossed in this book. You must keep busy reading, but I think whoever just hit your car totaled it. And the driver is speeding away! Can you believe that?

Don't look now, but the driver stopped down the street to check out the damage to his own car. You could probably run out and get their license number, but don't. Just keep concentrating on what you are reading. Your car is totaled by a hit-and-run driver who is parked just down the street, but you just keep busy reading.

"Don't look now," is the oldest hypnotic trick in the business. "Don't think about the position of your left foot… Don't notice that your left shoe is feeling tighter and tighter." What happens when someone tells you something like that?

And when we are faced with a major loss in our life, like the loss of a loved one due to death, and someone tells us—"Don't think about Bill (or Sue, or Aunt Mary, or Grandpa), just keep busy!" What are we likely to do? The only words we remember are think about Bill. That is what hypnosis is all about, and we do this every day to each other! We scream at our kids, "Don't run into the street!" And where is the first place they go?

We preach, "Don't be late!" "Don't do drugs!" "Don't have sex!" Look at the kids in our world today, and you can see how well this strategy works.

It works better if we are honest—

"You *can* have sex, but let me tell you how I feel about it. Let me try to help you understand the truth and the consequences of sex...."

"You want to do drugs? If you want to, I cannot stop you. But, I can tell you what I know about drugs...."

"If you come home late I worry about your safety and I won't get to sleep when I go to bed. If I don't get to sleep because I'm worried about you, I suffer. I don't like to suffer, so please don't come home late."

"You can't get your mind off Bill? I know, it's tough to accept the fact that Bill is dead. It hurts. I love you, and I don't want you to feel pain, but you do. All I know is, I miss Bill, too. And, I need a hug."

If we appear disorganized in our grief it is because we are organized toward one thing. We do not want to make big decisions, because it all feels like it is just too much for us. Well, it is! In our grief, life overwhelms us. That is why, when someone close to us is grieving a major loss, it is important that we help wherever we can, by pointing out the rocks. Often, that means helping the grieving make major decisions in their lives. We may be called upon to help the grieving organize their thoughts as they move closer to accepting the truth of their loss.

When a person is bereaved they will also appear to be very restless. We see that restlessness, that agitation and chaos; and maybe that is why our first advice is, "Just keep busy." Well, we all do some of our *best* work when we are restlessly busy doing other things, don't we?

If you have ever driven a car you are an expert on this. What is your mind doing when you are driving? "Oh oh— A corner coming. Better push the brake pedal 2 1/2 inches...The vehicle is now slowing...Brake another 1/2 inch...Now, turn the wheel a bit to the left...Lift the brake 1/2 inch."

No one drives like that! We do some of our best and probably safest driving when we are not actually *thinking* about every minuscule point of driving. We drive almost unconsciously. We leave our conscious mind open, so we are able to react to situations as they present themselves on the road.

But in the meantime our minds stay quite busy doing other things. If our minds are too busy, we may do strange things. Have you ever seen a person run a red light? Ever wonder how many times you have run a red light and not realized it? You may have, because consciously you were not behind the wheel driving. You were somewhere else entirely, thinking of something completely different that took concentration away from your driving.

Sometimes, when women have some thinking to do, they might clean. I have seen women clean everything in the house, and then start in on the garage. These women get busy when they have deep thinking to do. And, they do some of their best thinking when they are busy.

It is the same with men. When men have troubles on their mind, they too may get busy. They clean out the garage, organize all the tools, and then try to organize the closets. And when they get busy, they do some of their best thinking, too. When a person is grieving a major loss in his life, it is important not to say "keep busy," but rather, *"get* busy." Keeping busy will accomplish nothing. Getting busy on the job of grieving will help the survivor accomplish a lot. *"I know, it hurts! It's hard for you to concentrate on anything else. But, if you get busy, you can work through your grief."* Getting busy on your grief —recognizing what you have lost and how you feel about that loss— is a necessary task.

In most businesses when an employee experiences the death of an immediate family member, the business will give that employee some days off, with or without pay. And while we know that is a wonderful gesture on the part of the employer, the fact is, the employer also knows that the bereaved employee is not worth a damn on the job. They are usually unable, emotionally or physically, to do their job. The bereaved employee is also more prone to injury, and could be a source of accidents, because he or she will not be thinking clearly.

There is a lot of restlessness in the bereaved, and at times, restlessness is exhibited in pacing. Have you ever noticed how people have a tendency to pace in their grief? Pacing serves a real and important purpose. It is a way for the bereaved to act out the searching behaviors that often follow a loss.

Restlessness is a part of searching. Whenever we lose something, we search in an attempt to recover what we have lost. Just think about the search that goes on when you lose something as simple as your car keys.

Have you ever watched a man searching for his lost car keys? The man's search is very ritualistic. First, he pats all of his pockets: his front pant pockets; his back pant pockets; his jacket pockets; then, his shirt pockets. He will look at his still-empty, out-stretched hands with bewilderment.

Next, he will explore the depths and trinkets in each of those pockets: his front pant pockets; his back pant pockets; his jacket pockets; then, his shirt pockets. And again, he will look at his still-empty, out-stretched hands with bewilderment. Then he will start all over again: patting down his pockets; then, searching through his pockets; this ritual can go on for ten minutes.

Have you ever seen a woman searching for a lost pair of pliers? It is a very ritualistic process, as well. Her eyes will dart across the counter tops as she moves to one end of the counter. She opens drawer number 1. No pliers? So, she moves on to drawer number 2. Still no pliers? On to drawer number 3, then drawer number 4, and on and on to the last drawer.

If the woman does not happen to find the pliers, what does she do? She steps back to the end of the counter as her eyes dart across the counter tops. And then, she proceeds to search every drawer over again in the same ritualistic order she searched them the first time.

Whenever we lose something, we launch a formal or ceremonial process to search for what we have lost. You may know a person who has lost a spouse due to death, and in the middle of the night, that person will just go for a drive. The person will hop in the car, back out of the driveway, and steer as the car moves. Ask the person where his car took him, and he will answer, *"Oh, I don't know* —I just drove." Take out a city map and ask him to show you where he drove. Chances are, he drove by the restaurant he and his wife used to go to every Wednesday night. Or he just happened to drive by the place they both went to worship every week. And chances are very good that his drive took him by the cemetery where his wife is now buried.

Cry Until You Laugh

When a survivor searches for the person he has lost due to death, chances are that his midnight drive —his search— will eventually take him to the cemetery. Oh, it might be the long way of getting there, but he will end up there sooner or later. The sad thing is, most of our cemeteries are locked at night.

We may hear that the reason we lock our cemeteries at night is to keep kids from vandalizing the place. And while a couple of security guards stationed at the cemetery could do a better job than a high fence and locked gates, we would be hard pressed to find someone willing to work in such a capacity.

I think kids have a purpose in going to cemeteries at night. There, they can get close to death; they can sit on the graves, drink beer, turn over stones and emerge unscathed. "Ha Ha! See what I did? And *Death didn't get me!*" That can be an educational process. Kids need to learn that death is not lurking around the corner, waiting to get them. But, before kids feel a need to break into a locked cemetery, why don't we take them there on a school field trip? It might help them learn about the reality of death. Again, we do not, because that would be weird, unbelievable, and in bad taste.

Kids or adults, it doesn't matter how old we are, we all search. We search for the meaning of death. We search for ways to overcome death. We search in an attempt to regain what we have lost to death. And in our futile investigations we miss the more important search for life, what it means to be alive, and for ways to live before we die.

141

Where the search will take us, we aren't exactly sure. All we know is that we must search until we come to the full truth and reality of what it is we have lost. How we search is not as important as the result of the search. If we are ever to work through our grief, we will search in order to experience the fullness of our loss.

In that context, people have often asked me if I think it is healthy for survivors of a death to view the body of the dead, and I have always answered that it's not only healthy, it's imperative! "But Dick," someone will ask, "it was *suicide.* One *shotgun* blast to the head, you know. How can you expect the survivors to *view the body?*"

I respond, "What *part* of the body *can* the survivors view? Can the head be covered and the torso dressed and left uncovered?..."

"Well, we'll just put up a picture of the recently departed. That will be so much easier!"

Easier for *whom?* The funeral director? Or the family member that does not want to accept the fullness of the loss? Or the relative that does not want everyone to know the real nature of the death? *Who are we trying to fool?* Who are we hurting when we deny the fullness of a loss due to suicide? The questions become all too real three months after the funeral when one of the family is found searching a dark cemetery after having driven around town all night.

142

Cry Until You Laugh

If I happen to die in a car accident and the funeral director cannot show my face because of the nature of my fatal injuries, I would hope —for my grieving wife's sake— that the funeral director wraps my face in gauze and displays the rest of my body. I am confident that my wife would recognize my hands, my jewelry, or my clothes.

When survivors see the hands, the watch, the ring, any tattoos, scars, or familiar clothing —any kind of identifying marks— they begin to come to terms with the fullness of their loss. Part of the search can be over. The reality of the loss can begin to set in, and the remaining work of grief can commence.

A few years ago I became familiar with a family who had lost their father to drowning. The funeral director in charge of the arrangements made an initial, somewhat frantic call to me. He told me the family wanted to view the body and there was nothing that could be done to make the deteriorated body presentable. I suggested to this funeral director that he do whatever he could do, and then let the family view the body. He agreed on one condition —that I be there when family members arrived.

I arrived at the funeral home just as the family drove up. I could tell, as the individuals got out of the car, that some members of the family had been drinking heavily. In fact, an older man — presumably the man's brother— was quite drunk. As the family entered the funeral home, they began to gather in the back of the viewing room. The drunken man stumbled towards the open casket calling his brother's name over and over. As he stood by his brother's casket, he began to yell and curse. He cursed his brother, the police, the medics, and himself. Finally, he leaned over the open casket and touched his brother's body. He stopped crying, stopped cursing, and turned towards me. "Boy," he said, "my brother really looks dead, doesn't he?"

Even in a state of drunkenness, this man used all his senses to come to terms with what he knew he knew. He saw. He touched. He smelled. Now, he knew his brother was DEAD dead. Even though this man was drunk, he no longer had lingering questions about his brother being dead.

Some twenty years ago, I received a call from another funeral director who also wanted my help. This director told me that a mother had come to him and desperately wanted to see her son's body. The problem was, her son had been dead for 28 years and never buried! Apparently, the son had been shot down over a jungle in China in 1945, and the airplane and the body had been recently discovered.

I told the funeral director that I did not understand what the problem was. He responded, "Dick, that woman doesn't want to see the body. I know she doesn't."

I asked him if he had the body, and he told me he had portions of the body: a skull, humerus, and a few other small bones. And, yes, he had the man's dog tags. He commented, "She tells me she needs to see the body. But Dick, she doesn't want to see this body." I reminded him that he already told me that, but the fact was, the woman needed what she said she needed.

The funeral director believed that he knew what the woman wanted, but he obviously did not hear her tell him what she *needed.* And, in some cases, survivors may not *want* to view a dead body, but it may be something they desperately *need.* This woman said she needed to see her son's body. Who was I, who are we, to say any different?

Again, the funeral director agreed to show this woman the remains of her son, as long as I was there when it happened. I arrived at the funeral home before the woman, and the funeral director and I laid out the remains. I put the skull on the pillow of the casket, the miscellaneous bones in their respective places, and the dog tags right up front. When the woman arrived she proceeded directly to the casket that displayed these remains. She touched the skull, carefully moved her hand across one of the bones, and picked up the dog tags. She looked up to me and said— "Thank God, it's over. After 28 years, *it's finally over!"*

She told me that for 28 years, every time the doorbell rang, every time the phone rang, every time the mailman stopped by her mailbox —*every day* for 28 years— she thought she would hear from her son. And now, the waiting could be over.

We might understand why it is important for some to have the remains of those killed in Viet Nam returned to the United States. When you see pictures of families grieving beside the caskets that contain the remains of their brothers or fathers who have been missing in action for 22 years, you begin to understand that after 22 years, the survivors are still working through their grief.

Survivors of death will search until they come to understand the fullness of their loss. Searching is a part of working through grief. Searching is to be expected, but our society has a tendency to treat searching the same way we treat death; as weird, unbelievable, and in bad taste.

In a suburb of a large Midwestern community, a woman was arrested for trespassing in a cemetery. At 2 a.m., she had climbed the fence that surrounded the cemetery. The police saw a car parked near the fence and investigated. When they found the woman crying over the grave of her husband, they arrested her for trespassing. I just happened to be at the court house as the case was called, and I spoke to the judge. I explained to him why the woman might be in the cemetery at night. I told him that I thought we should unlock cemetery gates and provide security for survivors who have the need to search as they work through their grief. The judge spoke with the woman and dismissed the case.

A survivor does not have to be an immediate family member to have a need to search. Nurses will search when a patient of theirs has died. Have you seen that search take place? A nurse comes into work at 2 a.m. and someone says— *"So-and-so died last night..."*

146

Cry Until You Laugh

"No! *'So-and-so?'* Are you sure?" The first response is denial. "But, So-and-so was doing so well... You're *mistaken,* aren't you?" If death cannot be denied, then it must be a mistake. Soon, the nurse will comment, "So-and-so *really died,* huh? I told that dumb doctor to change those meds. If only he'd listened to me..." A little bit of blaming behavior and anger exhibited. Then you hear, "Wasn't anybody watching him? If only *I'd* been here, this never would have happened." Some anger directed at self; what society calls guilt.

Then, the nurse will get a queasy stomach, some *I've got-to-sit-down-a-minute* blues. Then there will be some disorganization, like: "...er, do I start in on my shift? Should I start with meds, or give baths, or...?" It is not long before that nurse meanders by her dead patient's room and glances in the door. Maybe the nurse will stop, push the door open a bit, and cautiously walk into the room. And, nine times out of ten, the bed will be empty. The dead body has already been moved down to the morgue. Or worse, another patient will already be lying in the bed.

And I don't envy the new patient. The nurse will feel some anger if there was any kind of relationship with the one who died. And, the anger may be directed toward the man or woman now lying in that bed. I have suggested to hospitals that they try to keep beds of a patient who has died empty for at least 24 hours. That 24 hours gives the staff —human beings who, by the nature of their work, have made tremendous investments in the lives of their patients— time to come to terms with the reality and fullness of the loss they

147

have incurred. Most hospitals tell me that they just cannot do that; it is not economically prudent.

Then I suggest these hospitals provide their staff with classes on Loss and Grief. I am told that nurses get plenty of instruction on death and dying in college —no need to talk about loss and grief, that's weird, unbelievable and in bad taste.

So nurses search. Doctors search. Volunteers search. These survivors may not know why —they may not even know that they do— but they search and ask why.

Why? A small word, with big significance. Members of the clergy hear that word a lot. "I just want to know, Pastor...Why? Why *my* child? Why *my* loved one? Why *me? What did I ever do* to deserve this?" And as these survivors search for answers, they often look to themselves. Those who believe that if they are good, they will receive good, may feel the death of a loved one must mean they are bad.

In his book, *When Bad Things Happen To Good People* (1981), Rabbi Herold Kushner makes the point that those who feel they are being punished for their past deeds are usually religious people. They often search through their past deeds with a religious microscope to discover some sin to explain why this bad thing happened to them. Of course, everyone will die at some point; our misdeeds or sins are not the cause of death. And it may help us in such a search to remember the fact that good things as well as bad things happen to all people.

Some of my favorite pictures are photos that show people searching near the Viet Nam memorial in Washington, D.C. You've seen the pictures of this memorial, America's own Wailing Wall. There are 58,022 names engraved in 275 stone blocks. Soon, our plans will include a monument to those Missing In Action. Why? Because we want to help survivors in their search for what and for whom they have lost.

If you have noticed, the Viet Nam memorial was designed to stand some feet apart from the walkway in front of the monument. Originally, there was a small strip of grass between the stone monument and the walkway. If you talked to Park staff, they would have said that little strip of grass was probably the most often replaced strip of grass in America. Today, the grass has been replaced by more stone. When someone goes to the wall to search for the name of a friend or loved one, no sliver of grass or florescent sign or barbed-wire fence will keep them from getting as close as they can to finding what they have lost; even if they only search for a name inscribed in black stone.

If you have ever gone to the monument, you know that you can actually get a map of the wall to help you locate the name of the person you are searching for. And, for most searchers, after they have found the name, they get a piece of paper, place it across the inscription and create a pencil rub or likeness of the name of the person they searched so hard to find.

We have all seen pictures of the men and women who go there to search for their buddies who died in the war. Many of the veterans who search this memorial do so in their camouflage uniforms, the kind of clothes they wore during the war. They know that when one is searching for a buddy, you should at least wear the kind of clothes your buddy could recognize.

It seems that we, as a society, always need stones when there has been a death. If there has been huge death, there will be huge stones. If many have died, there will be many stones. And, we will go searching at those stones. We will mourn at those stones. This searching happens even more often when the bodies of the dead have never been viewed. It is that way with the Viet Nam memorial. Many of those bodies were never seen by loved ones and survivors.

So we erect stones. Then we search those stones. We take rubbings of the inscriptions on those stones. And we take those rubbings home. Some people frame their rubbings and hang them in their homes so they will know their buddies have died. That is why we have always made cemetery stones from marble and granite. Those stones will be around forever, long after the memories of our buddies are gone.

When a survivor needs to search, he or she needs to know where to search. That's very important. It's one of the facts encountered by the survivors at a funeral. The trip to the cemetery can serve as the survivor's final search. So, the trip to the cemetery is an important part of working through grief. Except in some northern communities, where the weather is cold and the ground is frozen months at a time. There, you may find spring burials at the cemetery. Only a few close family members may be present, if even that, and many of the survivors never get the chance to experience the valuable lessons learned in the search that takes them to that final destination.

It does not even take frozen ground in some places to deny survivors the experience. "Oh, it's raining. Let's just conclude here at the church, or here at the funeral home. No need to go on to the cemetery." I hope funeral directors, clergy, and family understand that, for some, the search will not end there. For some, it just isn't over until it's finally over!

Detachment

Detachment is another place we will visit as we travel the road of working through our grief. This is an exhausting place, detachment. It is the place where we finally say, "Boy, I've had *enough* of this pain."

It is the point in our grief work when we exclaim, "I've gone through so much of this 'processing' stuff...I'm sick and tired of being sick and tired— I quit!"

Detachment is a lot like a taffy pull machine. You have probably seen a taffy pull machine before. The machine pulls at the candy, just about to the point where you think the candy will break, and then it wraps the taffy up again. Stretch and pull and fold, stretch and pull and fold.

The survivor says, "I'm tired of this pain. I quit," and then that song comes back on the radio to remind him of his wife.

"I've dealt with Dad's death, and I feel much better, thank you!" And then, she drives by Dad's favorite restaurant, and all the feelings come welling back up inside.

Just when you think you're all done with your divorce, he comes back to get the kids. And he *looks good!*

There may come a time in our detachment when we say to ourselves, "I'm sick of this." And so, we withdraw.

You have seen withdrawal. What happens in withdrawal is the survivor backs away. He backs away from other people; backs into her home; backs into his TV set; backs into the bedroom bringing her TV with her; backs into a bottle of booze and pulls the cork tight behind him. When people detach, they sometimes withdraw from churches, clubs, jobs and all social activity. People just withdraw, they back into themselves.

Health Care professionals know about drawing into oneself. If a patient is going through some painful treatment, doctors and nurses know that it is not a good idea to let that patient close his or her eyes during the procedure because then the pain is internalized.

When we feel pain, we have a tendency to pull inside, close our eyes, and wrap up in a tight little ball. We believe that means security. But, we actually need to do just the opposite. We need to open up when we feel pain; otherwise, there will be no place for the pain to go but in. Opening up reduces pain. Opening up allows us to get the pain out.

Traditionally, men have been notorious for withdrawing. We withdraw into our work. We work like crazy when we are feeling pain. It does not matter if we are physicians from Sheyboygan, janitors from Jacksonville, or preachers from Los Angeles, we will work like madmen all day long, have a couple of stiff jolts at night to help us sleep, and wake up the next day to do the same thing all over again. We believe that if we work hard enough, in six or eight months, we'll be over our grief. Plus, we'll get rewarded for all our hard work. We will make more money, maybe even earn a promotion and the praise of all our friends.

"Heh, isn't old Dick handling the death of his wife quite well? I mean, look at him. Only two weeks, and he's right back in the old saddle! Attaboy, Dick!"

And if that doesn't seem to work, we'll just increase the doses of withdrawal; the doses of work or of alcohol.

At the point of a major loss in our lives, some detachment can be quite healthy. The trouble comes when we put too much in front of the behavior. Working a little harder may be healthy (remember get busy), but working too much harder will create additional problems. Having a drink to help you sleep at night may be healthy, but drinking too much will create additional problems.

We can end up absorbed in ourselves, withdrawn to the point of no return. And all the while, we are putting off the work we will have to do if we are ever to process our grief.

When we see someone withdrawing into work or hobbies or drinking or any other behavior, we can only let them be aware of the rocks we see. We can ask ourselves if the behavior is typical for that person, given the circumstances of the loss they have incurred. We can ask ourselves how the increased behavior helps or hinders change in that person. Does it help or hinder that person as he or she tries to get in touch with reality?

One of the things I find terribly hard to do in my job as a counselor is to work with drunken little old ladies. I am seeing more drunken little old ladies than you can imagine. And each one of them is someone's grandma. It never gets any easier to talk to them or family members about their behavior. Still, more and more, widows are withdrawing into alcohol. Family members will tell me, "Dick, you're a nice man. And we certainly trust you. Everything you've said to us has been right on target. But Dick, you're wrong on this one. Grandma *can't* be a drunk!" All I am trying to do is point out a rock.

In the upper Midwest, people have a marvelous way of helping survivors deal with withdrawal. This has not been a hard topic to research, and even though the results of the research may be somewhat unscientific, the results are no less profound. People in the Midwest have what I call, the JELL-O Brigade.

Cry Until You Laugh

When someone is facing a loss due to death, the JELL-O Brigade get out their very best dishes —no cracks, chips, or dents in these dishes. They whip up their best salads, pies, cakes, cookies and casseroles, and take them to the bereaved. The JELL-O Brigade is very ingenious.

The JELL-O Brigade does two things. First, it force-feeds the family or survivors. I mean, these cooks don't prepare just one helping of goulash or two small pieces of cake for the family, they make a meal out of it. The survivor's counter is so full of dishes with pies and cakes and cookies; their refrigerator is so full of casseroles, desserts and home-baked breads, there is hardly room to store leftovers.

We know that the survivors of a death frequently tell you they don't need all that food. Oh, they'll say, they aren't hungry, that don't have time to eat, you shouldn't have gone through all that work, but they will eat what you bring them. Basic Midwestern values tell them they just cannot let all that food go to waste with kids starving in Ethiopia. And for the soldiers of the JELL-O Brigade, this ritual gives them the opportunity to extend their condolences, along with some compassionate, helping hands.

But something more important is accomplished by the JELL-O Brigade. Four days after the funeral, the widow is at home, sitting at the kitchen table, sipping a cup of coffee, praying to her God that she will die. "This is hell, Lord. I don't know how I'll live without him. Just let me die, too."

But after that prayer, she will look up from her steaming coffee, wipe the tears from her eyes, and it's like a bolt of lighting strikes her. She sees all those dishes —her friends' best silver trays, favorite casserole dishes, and precious crystal cake platters. Then she pleads, "Wait, Lord. Hold on just a minute. I can't die yet!"

The widow has to get those dishes back! She has probably already washed them clean, but will not recall when and how she did that. It doesn't matter. What matters is, the widow loads her friends' dishes into her car and personally returns them, one at a time.

And at every house, she begins, "Oh Joyce (or Betty, or Sue, or whatever), I don't know how to thank you. I just didn't have the energy to cook, and you were so thoughtful!"

"No problem. That's the least I could do. Can you come in for a cup of coffee?"

"Well, I have so much to do...I don't know... Well, I guess so —Just for a minute."

And the first thing the friend asks is, *"How are you doing?"* Up to now, the widow has been alone in her grief. Oh, her friends have visited. Her priest, minister, or rabbi stopped by every day. The kids came home and the relatives were there and she never seemed to be alone. In fact, for the past few days, it would have been difficult for anyone to have a private conversation with her. But now, she *talks.*

Cry Until You Laugh

She talks about her grief, her pain, her loneliness. "It's been hell. You just don't know, it's pure hell. Nobody else seems to understand. All of my friends still have their spouses. No one seems to be able to relate to me. Other widows are so much older, and I just can't relate to them. It's so empty around the house. I just can't seem to sleep in that bed. I sleep in the recliner every night. There are certain sounds in the house that drive me nuts. I think it's him. And there are certain smells that remind me of him, and I turn around, but he's not there. He's gone, isn't he?"

And she cries. She cries and these two friends hug each other and the coffee stands there getting cold. After an hour or two, the widow leaves because she has so many more dishes to return. And at every friend's house, she stops for coffee. And with every friend, she talks, she cries, she hugs. The friends just listen, offer soft shoulders and more hugs. And that is the best thing that could happen for the grieving widow —for anyone bereaved.

In big cities today, it seems that people just don't have time for the JELL-O Brigade. So, the bereaved go to therapists. And hopefully, the therapist helps the bereaved talk so they can hear themselves as they re-define who they are now, after their loss.

Some communities who still have the JELL-O Brigade are on the verge of muddling it up because friends are beginning to deliver food in disposable pie tins and on paper plates. Please don't do that! When you take food to survivors, use your best china, your best silver, your most precious dish, even the family heirloom.

You do not throw away family heirlooms; and you would not sell a family heirloom at any price. Don't worry, the bereaved will know how precious these dishes are to you. They will return them, personally.

And the bereaved will probably take time to have a cup of coffee, if you invite him or her in. He will re-tell the story of his grief over and over and over, as long as he has dishes to return. She will begin to come to terms with the fullness, the reality of her loss. Each time the survivors tell their story, they will cry and they will get comforted. And each time, the fullness of the loss will get easier and easier to accept.

One other word of caution. Don't ever offer to return dishes for the widows or widowers. Let them do that on their own, because there is method to the madness. Important healing happens. It helps end the survivor's desire to withdraw. And it accomplishes, in a very economical way, what might take months at a counselor's office.

Reorganization

As I've suggested, grief is a process whereby we—

☆ *identify the fullness of a loss we've incurred*
☆ *identify the feelings that result*
☆ *begin to re-identify who we are, after the loss*

At some point in grief, if the bereaved has worked through these areas, he or she will begin to exhibit some signs of re-identification, or *reorganization* of self.

The first sign is that the bereaved can talk out loud about the loss they have incurred. You will hear people say, "I got divorced." Or, "I lost a leg." Or, "My spouse died." Or, "My child died." The bereaved begins to verbalize the truthfulness of the loss. You actually hear the words "I" and "me" in the statements. You hear "divorced" instead of "separated." You hear "died" instead of "passed away." These words are a good sign of reorganization.

Sometimes the words come very quickly after a loss. Sometimes it takes awhile. But, when it begins, we know that the grieving have begun to reorganize their lives, or have begun to re-identify who they are now, after their loss.

Another good sign of reorganization is when the bereaved is no longer emotionally overwhelmed by the loss. It comes when the bereaved can talk about the fullness of their loss, and not become emotionally overwhelmed. Their world and their life is different now, but life *does* go on.

You might hear someone say, "My wife died. She had an illness, a terrible illness. I remember the day she died. I took her to the hospital, and..." And the survivor continues talking about the loss. You might see tears in the eyes or a lump in the throat while the survivor talks. And that might be six, or sixty years later. But, the bereaved is no longer overwhelmed by feelings.

Another sign is when the bereaved can talk realistically about the loss or the person who died. You know that after a death, a lot of saints are born. You have heard the bereaved talk about the dead: "Oh, he was a *perfect* husband, a great man. I'm telling you, there was no one kinder, more..."

A little while into the grieving process, you might hear, "Yes, he was a *wonderful* man..." You hear the description go from perfect to wonderful. Then a little more time (and hard work) passes, and you hear, "He was a *fine* man—" Then it's, "He was a *good* man, but I'll never forget the time he..." You begin to hear that the survivor was married to a full human being; that the marriage was somewhat less than perfect.

In loss due to divorce, you hear just the opposite. First, its, "Yeah, well I hope the sucker gets hit by a truck! I've always hated his guts, that no-good scum!" After a while, "Oh, we had a rotten marriage, all right. Things weren't that good. But, I'll tell you, he was good with the kids." All of the sudden, you hear the beginnings of reorganization when the words are, "You know, compared to some of the doorknobs I'm running into at those single meetings, So-and-so wasn't all that bad!" You hear the bad, the good, and the in-between.

Another good sign of reorganization is when the bereaved begins to feel good about feeling good. You know what I am talking about: there is a big difference between feeling good and feeling good about feeling good.

Cry Until You Laugh

I wish I had a videotape of my mother during the first few months after my father's death. You would be able to see how she began, slowly but surely, to feel good about feeling good.

About three months after my father died I asked my mother how she was doing. I could see her eyebrows tense up. Her lips drew tighter and she said, "I think I'm doing much better, now."

I asked, "Mom, why do you say that?"

She replied, "Well, it's like the other night. I was watching the *Carol Burnett Show* and that crazy Tim Conway did his old-man 'shuffle.' I was sitting there watching, and I started to laugh. Then I thought, Oh my God, it's only been three months..." My mother was coming to terms with the fullness of her loss, and she was beginning to feel better. But, it still wasn't O.K. to be feeling too good. It wasn't O.K. to laugh, just yet.

About nine months later, I again asked my mother how she was doing. She raised her eyebrows, smiled and said "Oh, I'm doing much better now. You know, just the other night, the gals and I went out for dinner. We played some bingo, drank a little wine, told a few stories, and I got the giggles. I didn't get home until about 11 o'clock. As I was getting undressed for bed, I realized that my sides hurt from laughing so hard. I sat there and said to myself, boy, that *sure feels good!*"

My mother said, "that sure feels good." There was a little

tear in her eye. There was some sadness in her voice. But, she felt good about feeling good.

When the bereaved can eat, taste, and enjoy the food they eat, that is a sign of feeling good about feeling good.

When the bereaved hears a song that reminds him of the person he has lost, a tear might come to his eye, but he still enjoys the song. When the bereaved walks in the park and hears a familiar bird calling and is reminded of the past, a smile comes to her face because she remembers good feelings she used to share with her loved one. The bereaved begin to feel good about feeling good.

You can really notice the beginnings of reorganization of self in relation to sexual behaviors —when the bereaved can feel good about feeling good sexually. Widows, in particular, do not like to talk about those feelings. In counseling, I will ask a widow how she is doing, and she will tell me, "Oh, I'm getting some of *those same feelings* back again."

I'll ask, "What feelings?"

She'll say, "Oh, Dick, *you know—*"

And I'll say, "No, I don't know. What feelings are you talking about."

And she'll smile, bow her head and say, "THOSE feelings."

Cry Until You Laugh

Well, that is a beginning; a sign that it is O.K. to feel good about feeling good.

You can imagine the problems sexuality creates in a relationship when a couple's child has died. Here are two bereaved people, a husband and wife, that will never be at the same place in their grieving. Both have different kinds of investments in the child they lost. Both have different ways and times of working through their grief. It is almost as if the husband and wife orbit each other in their grief. When one is down, the other is up.

One day, dad is down in sewer city with his grief, and mom does not want to go down there because she knows how painful it is. So mom stays away from dad. The next day, dad's up, feeling good about feeling good, and it is mom who's in the dumps. Ol' dad, he signals that he is ready for some affection, and mom says, *"Are you crazy?* Don't you know I'm hurting? How can you think about *sex* at a time like this?"

Mom and dad are bereaved. They are people in the midst of working through their individual grief, and are never in the same place. How many times in life are husband and wife in the same place emotionally when they are not grieving, let alone, in the throes of grief? Have you ever been with your spouse or partner at a time when your eyes meet, your hands touch and you both know it is time? So, you make mad, passionate love in the dining room at the Howard Johnson's. No, it does not work that way. Two people are seldom in the same place emotionally, at the same time.

Richard J. Obershaw, MSW, LISCW

In the midst of the pain of grief, a couple are often worlds apart. Mom and dad keep distancing each other in grief because they are not the same people they were before their loss. Mom and dad are *different* now —they have changed. And both are in the middle of re-identifying who they are now, after their loss.

We have to talk to these people about the changes that have occurred in their relationship, because they will have to talk about it. Mom and dad will have to confront themselves, as they are now, individually and within their relationship. Research shows that nearly 80% of all couples whose children die of leukemia are very close to divorce, or will actually divorce, within one year of their child's death. And that happens, in part, because of *unresolved* grief.

It's important for us to keep in mind that the bereaved couple are at different places at different times throughout the process of working through their grief. There are many intertwining circumstances that affect the process. We can best help these people when we point out the rocks we see as they work through their grief. We can remind them that while it is no simple process, they will be able to work out their relationship, and their grief, if they are willing to work at re-identifying who they are now, individually and as a couple, after a major loss.

As a friend of the grieving person, we can tell him or her about some of the rocks in the way. We cannot take away the pain. We cannot bring back what has been lost. But we can point out the boulders and obstructions he or she will confront. And, in the case of

164

the married couple, we can suggest to them that they talk about their sexual relationship —a very big part of who they are as a couple. We can suggest they see a counselor to help them do some sorting out when things become a problem.

Another good sign of reorganization is when the bereaved decides that old friends have become just that —*old friends*. You see the bereaved beginning to interact with new people in new clubs, new groups, and new organizations. Sometimes clergy get really upset because the bereaved moves to another place of worship. He or she may have a tendency to believe that the bereaved is leaving him or her, personally. In reality, often what the bereaved is saying is, "This old church won't let me be Sally Smith." The church wants the widow to stay "Mrs. *John* Smith," and it is too much work for the widow to constantly fight that.

At times, we have to take great care to distinguish between what we believe to be an action of anger or withdrawal, and what might be real growth. When people tell me right after the death of a loved one that they are leaving their church or synagogue, I ask them why. I ask them to tell me what leaving their place of worship is really about. I have to ask them if they are leaving because other members will not let them be the person they are now, or if it is something else entirely. I ask if they are leaving because they are angry at God or their rabbi, pastor, or priest.

Recently a woman I was counseling told me she was leaving her church. When I asked her why, she said that, for seven Sundays since her husband died, she went to the same early-morning service, sat in the same pew she and her husband had always sat in, and put the same amount of money in the collection. But not once had the pastor approached her, called her, or visited with her to talk about the death of her husband. All I could do was point out the rock. All I could do was ask her to talk to her pastor before she left her church. It could be that her pastor did not know she needed his support.

She came back to see me a couple of weeks later, and told me that she did talk to the pastor. "But," she added, "I probably could have done it in a better way." I asked her to explain.

She continued, "Well, last week, after the service, I went up to shake the pastor's hand, and said— "Nice sermon, pastor. By the way, did you notice Henry wasn't with me?"

Well, that worked for this woman. The pastor thought she was going crazy, so he gave her a follow-up call the next Tuesday and talked to her about her loss. He also explained the loss he felt. You see, the pastor was grieving, too. He was in a process of re-identifying who he was now because of the loss in his life. Here, the pastor had invested love, affection, kindness, and caring into his relationship with this woman's husband while he was dying, and he just did not want to be reminded of the loss. The widow and her pastor have a closer relationship now because they were both able to share the fullness of their individual losses.

I think there are times when the clergy should be sitting in the front row at the funeral with the family, instead of standing behind the podium delivering the sermon. Too often, the clergy have personal relationships with the dead, and they have to work through their grief as we all do.

Oftentimes, dating or re-marrying are signs of reorganization or re-identification. I caution survivors not to remarry for at least a year. I think that is sound advice. Re-identification takes hard work, and hard work takes time.

In addition, there will be many first events taking place — first birthdays, first anniversaries, first holidays— without the loved one. Each event will bring the widowed new realizations of new losses, new feelings that result because of those losses, and questions about who he or she is now because of that loss.

Many recently widowed or divorced people will redecorate their homes right after a loss. That can be a sign of re-identification of self. Divorced individuals often get rid of the bedroom set right away. Not always a bad idea. But, burning the bed? Now there's a rock!

Sometimes, the recently divorced will change curtains, furniture, kitchen cabinets. Sometimes, he or she will sell the house and move completely. I ask people to be cautious about making major changes really soon after a divorce, but they have to decide for themselves. The amount of change that can happen in a healthy fashion often depends on the seriousness of the loss.

You may have seen Holmes and Mashoeski's Social Readjustment Scale. All change and loss creates some amount of stress in our lives. Stress can be healthy, but it can also be a reason to withdraw. The purpose of the scale is to help identify stressors in your life. When you approach 300 on the scale, you are getting pretty close to being stressed out. Death of a spouse is rated 100 points, then values go down as you move down the list; a change in jobs, relocation, mortgages and other miscellaneous stressors are all allocated a number of points. When you get over 300 points on that scale, you are likely to get physically sick. This scale does a good job of pointing out rocks when we are confronted with stress from change or loss.

Tasks Of Mourning

J. William Worden states there are four major tasks of mourning that must be accomplished by the bereaved. These tasks are important to us as we help ourselves or others through grief. As we come to terms with the fullness of a loss, it is likely that we will accomplish all of these tasks.

The first task is to work to accept the reality of our loss. Society may want us to believe that the person has *expired, passed-on* or *bought the farm,* but the truth will be that the person is DEAD dead. At some point we will need to accept the natural law that tells us that person is gone and will never return; that reunion with that person in this life is impossible.

Cry Until You Laugh

With divorce, the state will tell us that the marriage is dissolved, we are married no longer. No longer are we separated, apart, or having disagreements, we are divorced. It will not help us to expect to receive a tax deduction, help around the yard, help with the dishes, or sexual gratification from our spouse. We are no longer married to him or her. The sooner we come to terms with the fullness of our loss, the sooner we can begin to re-identify who we are now, after the loss.

Anything you or I can do to assist the bereaved —no matter what has been lost— in accomplishing this first task will help them in their recovery from grief. For instance, talking about death, comforting the survivors, encouraging a truthful view of death, and remembering the death even weeks, months, or years from now, help the bereaved address the reality of their loss.

The second task is to experience the pain of our grief. Collin Murray Parkes stated, "Anything that continually allows a person to avoid or suppress the pain of a loss can be expected to prolong the course of mourning."

When we are grieving, we will try *anything* to avoid pain. We will avoid painful thoughts at all costs no matter how extreme the methods. One of my clients would masturbate every time the pain became too evident to him, and that was 20 to 30 times every day. People get into bizarre sexual relationships because they are trying to avoid feeling the full pain of their loss. It has little to do with sex, and more to do with trying to stop the thoughts that bring about the pain.

Richard J. Obershaw, MSW, LISCW

Another way we work at avoiding pain is to idealize the dead. It takes tremendous work on our part to portray the dead as a perfect saint. And in that hard work, we can avoid the pain. Conversely, we can work hard making a Devil out of the dead. *"No big deal. He was a real jerk, anyway...Doesn't bother me a bit that my friend died."*

We may move —the proverbial geographical cure— to avoid pain, but it does not work for long. We know it does not work for long, but we move anyway. When we move, we hope there will be fewer things to remind us of our loss, fewer things to cause us pain. The problem is that we take ourselves with us, and the pain of working through grief remains.

It is very important that we accept the task of experiencing the pain of our loss. It is imperitive if we are ever to work through our grief. The important thing is that we don't do it alone. Pain is something we should share with others because that is a healthy way to work through the pain.

The third task we will encounter in our mourning is to adjust to our new environment. When we lose something close to us, our whole world seems to change. Things are not the same any more. Part of our job will be to recognize what we have lost, what our environment is like after our loss, and how to deal with that new environment.

It is easier to withdraw, to pull into ourselves, rather than face this new world. But if we try to shrink the scary environment of our grief, we will cease to grow. We need to try to see the world from a broader perspective, a view that will ultimately expand ourselves.

The fourth task we will confront is perhaps the hardest. That task is to withdraw the emotional energy we have invested in the person or object we have lost; and then to reinvest that energy in someone or something else. That is difficult, because we know that if we reinvest our energy, we may be setting ourselves up for another loss and more pain. And quite possibly, more work through more grief.

So we hear the divorcee say, "Never again! Never EVER again, will I get married." It just means too much pain. After a relationship ends in divorce, it is easy to imagine there is just too much hurt in marriage. But, the reality is, all relationships will end.

All jobs will end. All health will end. All life will end. If we fail to come to grips with the reality of these facts, we may never come to appreciate the reality of those relationships, those jobs, that health, or our lives!

When we lose something we love —be it a person, place or thing— we come to a clearer understanding of the relationship we had with what we loved; and consequently, we come to better understand ourselves. That understanding can only be accomplished by work, by healthy grieving.

Unresolved grief prohibits us from making new investments in relationships. We know what we know! "If I invest again, I will lose. And if I lose again, I will have to face more grief. That would overwhelm me; I just can't do it again!"

When we are confronted with a loss, the goals are to—

    ★   *complete the tasks of mourning*
    ★   *to accept the reality of our loss*
    ★   *to experience the fullness of feelings*
            that result from our loss
    ★   *to adjust to our new environment*

Through reading, counseling, friends, grief-groups, or prayer, we can gather the strength and support we need to work through our loss and grief.

chapter five

The Myths of Grief

Definition of a Myth. The Myths. The Problems Associated with These Myths.

When we, or people we care about, are grieving a loss, painful feelings result. It is only natural for us to want to avoid pain. If we believe that someone we care about is experiencing pain, it is natural for us to want to help minimize the pain for him or her. But no matter how much we want to avoid pain, no matter how compassionate our motives are to help someone we love avoid pain, we do more harm than good when we try to do so by perpetuating what I call the *Myths of Grief.*

I have taken it upon myself, for over ten years, to do what I can to erase these myths. I get so far behind that sometimes I believe I'm leading a futile crusade. If we ever hope to dispel the unhealthy untruths about death and grief, or if we ever hope to help ourselves or others work through grief, we can begin by working to eliminate the myths of grief.

Definition of a Myth

Earlier, we attempted to define the word death. We searched for the meaning of the word; we asked ourselves when is somebody dead; and we looked at society's feelings about death and grief.

Once again, I turn to *Webster* to define the term myth. MYTH is defined as "a popular belief or tradition that has grown up around something." We all know that most popular myths are simply not true. And if believed to be true, cause confusion, fear, more pain and more misery than necessary.

I have already stated that I believe our society perpetuates many myths about grief. And as you read earlier, society does the same thing with death. When someone dies and society says that person passed on or expired, we are only avoiding the inevitable truth. We do that, in part, because of our fear of death and our feeling of powerlessness over death. If we, as individuals, can't conquer death or control the force it has over us, we will do whatever we can do to avoid it, to withdraw from it, or deny it. There is strength in numbers, so we do this as a society.

Pain and suffering often accompany grief. While we can work through the pain and overcome the suffering, it requires hard work, and it seems easier to avoid the truth and hide ourselves behind the false security of our myths. The more people we can get to support us in hiding, the more power we believe we have over the truth.

Well, the pain, suffering, and hard work that accompanies grief cannot be avoided. Though we may try at all costs, all we do is create problems and compound the pain, the suffering, and the work that will be necessary.

Let's look at some of the myths of grief—

"Time Will Heal."

What a terrible lie! And we hear it all the time. A widow stands tearfully in the back of the church and a well-intentioned friend walks up and says, *"Don't worry, Jenny. Time will heal!"*

Cry Until You Laugh

Can you tell me one thing that time has ever healed?

How about a cut on your finger? Does time heal that cut? Cut your finger tomorrow morning while you are slicing a bagel and just don't do anything about it. Wait for time to heal it. Don't wash it. Don't put antiseptic, a BAND-AID, or ointment on it. Don't give that cut any kind of care and let time take its course. Will your cut heal?

If you're walking to your car after work, and stumble and break your leg, do your friends walk by and say, "Yo, Fred! Nasty break, you got there... Bone's sticking out... Blood gushing all over the pavement. Looks like you're in a lot of pain. But, don't worry Fred, time will heal!" That would be ridiculous!

Nurses, doctors and even mothers can tell you, time will not heal a broken leg. Infection might set in. Gangrene could result. A person could die of a broken leg, if he or she waited for "time to heal" it. Of course, there are those who would remind me that, yes, bones can heal themselves, if left alone for some time. But a bone left to heal itself will seldom heal properly. A person could be handicapped, and quite possibly in pain, for the rest of his or her life.

When people have broken bones, someone has to work to get them to the hospital. Someone has to work to clean the wound. Someone has to work to set the bone. Someone has to work to immobilize the leg. Then, after a period of hard work on the part of the patient to stay off the broken leg, someone has to work to take off the cast. Then, the patient may have weeks or months of strenuous physical therapy —more work.

What it takes to heal a broken leg, a cut finger, or the pain and suffering due to a loss in one's life is hard work. And after all that work, somebody's going to say, "Boy, time sure healed that broken leg!" Not true! *Hard work* healed that broken leg.

While speaking a few years ago in Michigan, I asked my audience to name one thing that time heals. A man yelled out, *"Pregnancy!"* Every woman in the place looked at that man as he sank lower in his chair, and then one woman shouted, *"Labor healed that!"* Yes, labor! Now, I can't speak from experience, but a mother can tell you whether or not labor is hard work. I'd bet it is!

Time won't heal grief, either. Hard work heals grief. The grieving have to work hard to—

    ☆   *identify their loss*
    ☆   *identify the feelings they are experiencing*
            as a result of their loss
    ☆   *re-identify who they are now, after their loss*

When you tell the bereaved that time will heal, the first question they will often ask is, "Well, how much time?" We may hear that it takes about a year to heal most grief, and some actually believe 365 days is what fixes you.

In this society, we have what I call the 13-month "wonder

widow." Have you ever seen her? She believes and professes that in one year she'll be over the loss of her husband. Everyone tells her that in a year she'll be done with the pain and the suffering. One year goes by and the widow is not only not better, she's feeling worse. So, the widow will tell herself, "thirty more days. I'll give it thirty more days, and then I'll be fine."

That's when I start seeing them in my office. After about 13 months of letting time heal the pain and the suffering, they come to my office ready to go to work on their grief. At grief groups you'll see 13-month wonder widows appear out of the woodwork. *"It's been over a year and I know I should be all better, but I'm feeling worse,"* and the only work they've done is pull sheets off the calendar.

With divorce it's the same. A lot of divorced people remarry as soon as possible after that first year has passed. At least after one year it's O.K. for them to have intimate relationships again. Or, now that one year has passed, they can go ahead and sell the house or kick the kids out or change jobs. It does not matter whether or not they have worked on re-identifying who they are now, after their divorce. The main thing to them is the amount of time that has passed. They think one year should be enough time, so now, they can get on with life. It does not matter if they have gained any new skills or strengths, and as a result, many go on to repeat some of the same mistakes that led them to the painful situation of divorce in the first place.

Richard J. Obershaw, MSW, LISCW

Recovering alcoholics hear, "Don't make any important decisions for the first year of continuous sobriety. Then after a year, you can, because you'll be better." Sometimes, the first momentous decision the recovering alcoholic makes on his or her one-year anniversary is to go get drunk. For one year, the pain has been unbearable. A year has gone by, and the alcoholic has gone to meetings listened to a lot of stories, but the pain just hasn't gone away because all the person has been doing is collecting anniversary medallions at 30 days, at three months, at six months, and now, at one year. There has been no hard work to re-identify who he or she is now, after losing the beloved companion, alcohol.

In at least one large mid-western community, there is a bar that gives free drinks to alcoholics in trade for their one-year anniversary medallions. That bar knows if the recovering alcoholic has not been doing anything but waiting for time to heal the hurt and pain, he or she will be back.

"A year, and you'll be better; you'll be fine," is just not true. In a year, if you work hard. In six months, if you *work hard*. In a year and a half, if you WORK HARD. It depends on what you had invested in what you lost, and how hard you work to re-identify who you are now, after that loss. The time involved has nothing to do with the grieving or the healing process. How hard you work during the time determines how soon, and to what extent you process your grief.

I know of a woman whose husband killed their three children and himself. In six months, the woman had processed the majority of her pain. She worked very hard at it; she spent four hours a week in therapy working through her pain. But her family couldn't accept her recovery. She wasn't supposed to be O.K. for a year or more, so the entire family ostracized her and pushed her away because they believed she must be crazy.

They thought she didn't grieve *long enough*. Who do you think had the problems working through their grief, the woman or her family?

If you truly want to help the grieving, or help yourself when you are grieving, don't say or believe that "Time Will Heal." It is a myth. *The reality is hard work heals*. The bereaved will need time to do their grief work, but time alone won't heal.

"You'll Get Over It."

In the midst of grief you will often hear someone say, *"Don't worry. You'll get over it."* That's another lie. The fact is when you experience a loss in your life you will *never* get over it. You will never be the same person you were before the loss. You may work hard through your grief, but you will never be the same.

Do you recall the first love in your life, your first boyfriend or girlfriend? You probably still have memories, thoughts and feelings for that person. Some of us can still recall those *good ol' days....*

Recently I was in Omaha, Nebraska, and I happened to see

181

the person that was the first love of my life. I recalled many of the details and feelings I had on our first date—our first kiss, our first—...you get the idea. All those memories came back to me vividly. Imagine yourself at your high school reunion, seeing some of your old buddies and friends again. When all the feelings come up to your throat, when the tears start to flow and you don't feel right because you thought you were over all those old relationships, don't worry because you aren't over them. They are still a part —and maybe a very important part—of who you are today.

For widows or widowers, years can pass, and they'll think they *should* be over their loss. Then a song will play on the radio, or they will drive by that old, familiar restaurant, or they will glance at somebody walking down the street with an old, familiar jaunt. The pain will start in the stomach and go up to the throat and the tears will flow, and they might think that something is wrong with them because they believed they should be "over" their loss by now.

When you see people in that condition, tell them it's O.K. Tell them they will never get over their loss. Give them, at least, the relief of knowing that *they are not going crazy.* When someone whose father died ten long years ago talks to you about Dad and the tears start to flow, don't think there's something wrong with him or her. See those tears as the result of some genuine love and compassion and some real pain due to loss. Then, give the support and love the person so well deserves.

The statement, "You'll get over it," is a myth. The truth is, you can work hard through the grief, but you will never get over the loss.

"This is Just a Stage You're Going Through."

Some of us have read about the stages of grief, those little points all in a row that we will go through as we grieve. Not true. There are no stages to grief.

I have already stated that grief is a process of working through the feelings that result from a loss. It is a process, not a program of step-by-step stages to recovery. If you believe that processing grief goes in stages, then it's easy to just sit around and wait for the next stage to come. People often use stages as events that they expect will happen to them —as if they have no control or power in the situation. Consequently, they feel more helpless —and hopeless— in their grief.

Have you ever seen that happen to a grieving person? They are in the throes of pain from the loss of a loved one, and they would just as soon stay right where they are because they are certain, "this too shall pass." But, grief will not pass if you sit and wait. It will take work.

Also, if you believe in stages of grief, and six months from now, you are angry again because of something you lost today, you'll think you're regressing. "Oh, my God! I'm going backwards! I'm not getting any better, I'm getting worse!" The fact is, you may have just recognized a new loss in your life, and with that new loss, new feelings and new work will be necessary to re-identify yourself within that loss.

The idea that grief happens in stages is a myth. The reality is, grief is a complex process that embodies a variety of feelings and behaviors. These feelings and behaviors are very much a part of the natural process of grief. As we work through grief, we may be at many, even concurrent places, in that process.

"True Believers Don't Cry."

This is a myth you may hear often when facing a loss, especially a loss due to death. As a result of the loss, the bereaved feels pain; and as a result of that pain, the bereaved mourns. The mourning is exhibited in tears. Then at the funeral, the pastor in the pulpit or a parishioner says, "No need to cry. If you are a true believer, this is a time of joyous celebration!"

Regardless of your religious beliefs, to suggest that *"true believers don't cry"* is to perpetuate a terrible myth. The myth suggests that if you are a true believer, if you have faith, you don't have to grieve. And if you mourn your loss by crying, you are then put in a position of having to grieve your loss of faith as well. There is something each of you can do to stop this myth where it starts. The next time you are at a Christian funeral and hear a priest or minister say, "No need to cry. No need to mourn this death," I want you to stand right up, and say, "Excuse me, pastor. . ."

The pastor will respond, "Yes, what is it?"

You continue, "Excuse me, pastor, but I am confused." Now, clergy hate for people to be confused. They will clarify their point until the proverbial cows come home. So the pastor will respond, "Well, what are you confused about, my dear?" And I want you to ask, "Pastor, what is the shortest sentence in the Bible?"

Few people at the funeral will know the answer, but don't worry, the pastor will. The pastor will know that the shortest sentence in the Bible is John 11:35— JESUS WEPT.

Jesus wept at the loss of His dear friend, Lazarus. This wasn't His dad, His mom, or His child, just His *friend;* and the kicker was, Jesus knew He'd get His friend back. Still, He wept as a result of His loss.

As you are sitting back down in the pew, tell the pastor, "Well, that's what confuses me, pastor. Rumor has it, that Jesus was a true believer!" You won't make many friends that way, but you will get the point across. To mourn the loss of a loved one *doesn't* mean you lack faith. Crying is a natural, healthy response to grief.

You do not hear the myth, "True believers don't cry,' spoken only at funerals. You hear someone say, "Don't cry—" you can always get another job, another spouse, another car, another what-ever. That is just another way for someone to say, "Don't grieve!"

"Anticipated Grief is Easier to Handle."
We do not hear this myth in such imposing words, but we still

hear it; only the words are, "long-term illness means short-term grief," or "Gee, you've known he was dying for six months. You should be prepared for his death."

You have heard it one way or another before. Sometimes it sounds like, "You're *lucky,* your wife is dying of cancer. My wife left all of the sudden —heart attack. The family had no time to prepare for her death!"

For a moment remember the diagram of *The Sequential Reactions To Loss* from page 112 of this book. And then imagine this scenario: The ambulance staff drives like crazy to answer a call to a private residence. When they arrive, a woman confronts them, *"Where have you been?* I called one half-hour ago!" Right away, you see the anger.

The medics rush into the room where the woman's husband lies quiet. An initial exam detects a faint pulse and shallow breathing. "Looks like a stroke," one of the medics tells the other. The woman yells, "He didn't have a stroke! My God, he's only 39 years old! Don't you guys even know how to do your job?" A little denial. A little more anger.

The woman wants to ride with the ambulance to the hospital. She appears confused as she hurries to find the green shoes that go with her green purse. Her stomach is upset, she's trying to get the dog secured in the basement, kids are crying in the other room —the woman appears very disorganized.

Cry Until You Laugh

Already this woman is feeling the loss of what was a healthy husband only moments ago. She's experiencing emotions associated with that loss, and she is mourning by displaying her emotions outwardly. In ignorance, one medic says to one another, "Got a 'difficult' woman here."

When the ambulance arrives at the hospital, the nurses and doctors work to stabilize the patient in the emergency room. The family gathers to wait, and one of the sons says, "What do you mean, I can't go in there and be with my dad? What kind of crazy rules do you have around here? I know the medic said stroke, but my dad couldn't have had a stroke. He was perfectly healthy the last time I saw him!" Some denial. Some anger.

But, the family waits. It's likely that the men pace, and the women huddle around mom and cry. The fullness of the loss of a healthy husband and father is beginning to be felt by all family members. In the meantime, you hear one nurse say to another, "They're going to be a difficult group, so watch them —especially the wife!"

The man is stabilized and is taken to the Intensive Care Unit. Here the family and hospital staff are at odds again. In this ICU only one person can spend five minutes of every hour with the patient, and that is at a distance. So it is the wife who visits her husband, but at best, from a great emotional and physical distance.

In a matter of days the woman has the entire hospital staff

upset. She's been to administration to tell them what she thinks about the hospital's rules— "If I could spend 55 minutes with him every hour, instead of just 5, he'd be better by now!" She's complained to the staff about her husband's care— "What do you mean, he can't even have plain water? You don't have to be a nurse to tell he's thirsty." And, she's complained to the doctor about her husband's illness— "If he didn't have to use a bedpan, if he could just get up and walk around a little, if he could just..."

A few weeks go by and the man has been moved to a private room. By now the wife is experiencing all kinds of physical symptoms and she's seeing her doctor about stress. She's not going to work. Her normal, everyday activities are all messed up. She's living in and out of the hospital, from a suitcase, sleeping in a chair in her husband's room. Her life is completely disorganized. And now the whole hospital staff is saying, "Whew! *That's* a 'difficult' woman!"

After some weeks in the hospital, the woman's husband dies. The doctor approaches her in the waiting room and says, "Mrs. So-and-so, I'm sorry. But your husband just passed away." The doctor cannot even say dead or died; he'll say "expired," "didn't make it," or "passed away." And the woman will respond, "No! No! That *can't* be true! Yesterday, he was doing so well! Tell me it isn't so..." And when the doctor says, "I'm sorry. But, there was nothing we could do," he has to watch his back-side! Some doctors have been hit, kicked, slapped, punched, and sworn at. When doctors tell survivors of the death of a loved one, they may see very angry behavior directed at them.

So, the woman will cry, and she will blame the hospital, the doctors, the nurses and God. "Dumb hospital. Dumb nurses. I should never have brought him here in the first place." Or, "Damn God! He was so healthy, so young. He had every reason to live, and *no reason to die!*" The wife will be disorganized, angry and full of denial.

But now, instead of "difficult woman we've got here," you hear the hospital staff being supportive. The nurses will put their arms around this woman. One nurse will get her a sweater. One nurse will call up family and friends. One nurse will get her a cup of coffee, etc.

Now this woman who displays some of the same behaviors she did before, does not get a "D" for DIFFICULT; she gets a "G" for GRIEVING. Now the woman is identified as grieving so the hospital staff comforts her. But the woman and every other family member has been grieving from the very beginning. When the ambulance took the man away from his home, they began grieving.

What did the woman lose when the medics first took her husband out of the house? She lost companionship. She lost her bed-partner. She lost the security of having a healthy husband. These were big losses. It stands to reason there was BIG grief.

What did the woman lose while her husband was in the

emergency room? She lost control! Do you grieve when you lose control? You bet you do! She lost a sense of security. She no longer knew what was going on with her husband, or herself She lost time with her spouse. These were all tremendous losses. The result was tremendous grief.

In intensive care the husband had wires connected to him, tubes coming out of his arms and his throat. He couldn't communicate well. Then, he had to squeeze once for yes, twice for no. Again, the woman experienced new and significant losses. There was new and significant grief.

And weeks later when the man died in his hospital bed, this woman lost hope for his recovery. All of the earlier loss was compounded by her husband's death, and the grief became even bigger.

With divorce you hear people say, "The hearing in court? Gonna be a breeze! Why, I kicked him out six months ago. It's been five months since I filed for divorce. The hearing only makes it all final. I knew that our relationship was over long ago!" However, when the judge slams the gavel on the bench and says, *"Divorce granted—"* people faint. Their legs don't work. They forget where they parked their cars. They cry and they curse and they blame. And they say, "My God! I thought I was over this thing." People who have been through divorce will tell you, because they know; you're not divorced until you are divorced.

Cry Until You Laugh

It's the same thing with death. A person's loved one is not dead, until he or she is DEAD dead.

It could have been six weeks or six months since the medics first took that man to the hospital, but now the widow is at the funeral home. She's crying, caressing the body of her dead husband, hugging family and friends, and some people say, "For heaven's sake, look at her! I mean, it's been six months. She knew her husband was dying. And here she is, crying and acting up. No, don't put your arm around her, you'll just encourage her! Besides, she should be past this stage by now!"

At the funeral home, what does this woman lose? She loses denial. She can no longer deny the death of her husband. She loses the ability to communicate with her husband, no more hand squeezes, yes or no.

Two days later at the cemetery, her husband's body is lowered into the grave; what does she lose? She loses the body of her husband. She's never going to see her loved one again. And later there will be that first anniversary without her husband, that first holiday without her husband, that first birthday without her husband.

All the woman's losses are tremendous losses. All mean tremendous grief. And in her mourning, people will suggest that she is just acting weird, unbelievable, or in bad taste because there was a long-term illness, and she had plenty of time to come to terms with her loss.

Richard J. Obershaw, MSW, LISCW

A few years ago I received a strange phone call in the middle of the night. I picked up the phone and a husky voice asked, "Is this the death man?"

Death man? I had been called worse things in my life, but death man was a first. I asked the caller what was on his mind and he explained, "I just got off work and drove by my mom's house. I noticed the light was on, so I stopped. I found my mother crying. She said she'd been crying for two days! She hasn't slept. She hasn't eaten. She's just been crying. I don't know what to do!" I asked him what his mother was crying about and he said, "I don't know. I didn't ask her. But Dad died six months ago. Maybe she's still upset about that."

I asked him to put his mom on the phone to talk to me. I told her that her son said she had been crying for two days. She said she had. "That sounds like a long time to be crying," I said. "What have you lost?"

This woman told me that she woke up two mornings ago and realized for the first time she couldn't remember the *sound of her husband's voice* anymore. Tremendous loss, tremendous grief.

Whenever you lose something, you will grieve. The woman had lost the ability to recall her husband's voice. That was a major loss to her, so she was experiencing major grief. Her son did not understand that because he imagined that she should be "over" her grief by now.

Cry Until You Laugh

If you believe that "anticipatory grief is easier to handle," tell me why parents of kids with leukemia have such tremendous grief when their children die? Those parents should be "all grieved out." They couldn't get a better chance to work through their grief; it's often four, five or six years of illness before the child's death!

Grief just doesn't work that way. When you perpetuate the myth that long-term anticipation of a loss makes grief easier to handle, you are maintaining a lie. Rather, when you or someone you know is mourning, ask, "What has just been lost?" When people tell you, "Oh, I must be crazy. I thought I'd be all grieved out by now," ask them what it is they have just realized they have lost?

One thing that long-term, anticipated loss can do is give survivors tools they can use to deal with losses as they occur. If survivors identify losses along the way, come to terms with the fullness of these losses, and re-identify who they are after the losses, they may be better prepared —physically, emotionally and spiritually— to accept other increasingly significant losses which occur. When we work through the pain and suffering that results from loss, we gain experience and tools to help us in the future. But, believing that long-term, anticipated loss is easier to handle allows us to withhold support and caring from the bereaved, because we believe that the survivors should be over it.

A closer-to-home example can be found in today's corporate culture. When people are given notice that their position within the company is being cut in six months, we figure they have plenty of time to grieve. "Gee Bill, I don't know *why* you're so upset. You've known for six months that your job was being cut! How come you're crying in your beer now?"

Long-term, anticipated loss is not necessarily easier to accept nor to work through than immediate, unexpected loss.

The idea that anticipated loss is easier to process than sudden, unexpected loss is a myth. The reality is, a lingering illness before a death, or long-term notice before a loss, doesn't make the loss any easier to accept when it finally does occur.

"All Death Means Loss."

Another myth would suggest that *all death means loss,* and that subsequently, grief will certainly follow that loss. This myth is expressed whenever we suggest that all loss must mean some pain. As a therapist I often administer a standard test that is designed to assess the emotional condition of my patients. The test is called the *Minnesota Multiphasic Personality Inventory,* or MMPI.

Like many other therapists, I give my patients this inventory on their first visit to my office. In a sense, this tool tells me how emotionally stable or unstable a patient is at that particular time.

The MMPI has more than 500 true/false questions for the patient to answer. The results of the test are plotted on a graph that shows levels of depression, states of obsessive/compulsive feelings or behaviors, anxiety, nervousness, introverted or extroverted characteristics, degree of honesty, and on and on. In the hands of a competent professional, this test is an important tool for therapists and patients alike.

In my lectures I show the audience the results of an MMPI from a woman who came to see me a couple of years ago. She came to see me for marriage counseling, and she brought her husband along. Both took the MMPI.

The results of the woman's MMPI showed me that she was depressed, anxious, fearful, disorganized, and very introverted. The results of her husband's MMPI gave me a hint to the reason; he was one of the most angry, chauvinistic, mean, hateful, inhuman humans I had ever come across.

The couple continued with counseling, and even I had a hard time sitting in the same room with this man. After three visits to my office, I found myself thinking, "When will this lady see the light? When will she see this man for all that he is, and leave this rotten relationship?" Certainly, I'm a counselor, but I am also a human being. It was obvious to me that the best thing this woman could do would be to end her marriage. However, I did stay objective, and I never let my opinion be known to either of these patients. In most counseling situations, it is important that clients identify and come to terms with their own perception of reality, or the steps necessary for their recovery.

I knew counseling was difficult for both of these people. The woman was coming to understand the man she had married, and the man was coming to terms with her growing awareness. As a result, he called off counseling and forbade his wife to ever see me again.

The following spring I received a telephone call from the woman. When I picked up the phone, she was very angry because she had been arguing with my secretary. At the time I wasn't taking any new patients, and she insisted that she needed to see me as soon as possible!

I imagined that this woman had finally made a decision about her insufferable marriage. Maybe there was hope after all! I offered to see her at the first available time on my calendar and asked if her husband would be coming in with her. She said, "Dick, didn't you hear? My husband *died* last February. He had a massive heart attack."

She went on to say that was why she wanted to see me. She said, "I know you do marriage counseling, but I also know you work with grief. And Dick, my grief just doesn't feel right!"

Well, when she came to my office, I gave her another MMPI. Her first MMPI showed her to be depressed, anxious, fearful, and disorganized. Now her MMPI showed her to be optimistic, very self-confident, and extremely calm.

So how did she spell relief? D-E-A-T-H.

✐

Cry Until You Laugh

When this woman lost her husband, she gained her mental health. She was still experiencing grief, but she was grieving the loss of the mental illness she carried through her marriage. She lost that illness with the death of her husband.

You know the grief associated with having to give up a physical illness if you have ever had a serious ankle, leg, or arm injury. When I came back from Viet Nam, I was on crutches. I found that everyone opened doors for me. People would talk to me and ask me about my injury. People would help me up stairs, carry my groceries to my car, and even caution others of my approach. *"Hey, move it up there! Got a man on crutches coming through!"* Even the parking attendant at my doctor's office helped me locate a convenient parking place. The day the doctor told me I could give up crutches, I was, at first, quite pleased. But as I rode the elevator down to the lobby, no one said a word to me. No one opened any doors for me. No one asked me how I was doing, or what happened after or wished me luck....

You may have known someone who has had a physical illness and wanted to hang on to that illness. People do not like the idea of having to work through the grief to re-identify who they are now, after the loss of their illness.

There are many widows who, after the deaths of their husbands, are heard to say, "I can finally eat the foods I want to eat. I can cook when I want to cook. I can go where I want, when I want." That doesn't mean that these widows don't still miss their spouses. But, they may realize some gains in the midst of their loss, even when that loss is due to death. When we perpetuate the myth that all death means only loss, we expect people will only feel sadness, and not happiness or relief We need to help the grieving understand that it is not wrong to feel some gain at the time of a loss. Otherwise, the grieving begin to think that there must be something terribly wrong with them, and that is not necessarily true.

To believe that all death means loss is to believe a myth. The reality is, when a relationship is empty, cruel, or abusive, death may not mean only the pain and suffering we often associate with grief. Death of a tormentor may actually result in feelings of joy or relief for the tormented.

"All Gain Means Happiness."

We hurt more than help when we perpetuate the myth that *gain means only happiness.* As a result, a new father or mother thinks he or she must be crazy to feel sadness at the birth of a child. Yes, the couple gains a child, but what do they lose? Maybe freedom. Maybe privacy. Maybe their sense of economic security. Maybe each other. When you become a parent, you lose your spouse; at least, everything that person used to be to you, including all of the attention your spouse used to direct just to you! A child is a big gain; but there can also be big losses associated with that gain.

Earlier, I suggested that if you experience what is perceived to be gain by society's standards, it is expected that you will only feel positive feelings, like happiness, delight, joy, and fascination.

Again, I use the example of winning a multi-million-dollar-mega-bucks-bingo-lottery. If such were the case, all of your friends would expect you to feel only happiness. There would be no more worries for you. You would have financial security for the rest of your life. You could have a new house, new car and new lifestyle. Winning the lottery would be a big gain for you. But it could also be a big loss because you might just lose your job, your present lifestyle, and the security of knowing who your real friends are!

Once, when speaking to a group of professional social workers, I suggested to my audience that they all worked in a job where people were experiencing loss and grief. A pretty young woman in the front row patiently raised her hand. One woman out of six hundred social workers in the audience, and this woman is in the front row to rebut my suggestion.

I asked her if she had a comment and she said, "Yes, Dick. I need to tell you, you are wrong on that point." I asked her, how I was wrong? She said, "I don't work with people facing loss and grief. I work in adoption. With adoption, there is only happiness."

Can you understand why I do not make that suggestion to groups of professionals anymore? My problem then was the need to dispel the myth that, in the case of adoption, there is only gain, and not loss as well.

Research suggests there is tremendous maternal deprivation felt by babies who are put up for adoption. And, I have to ask, *what loss is experienced by the mother or father who gives up their child for adoption?* I have to ask about the loss a couple feels when they have been childless for 15 years, but now have an adopted son or daughter. Some would believe that in adoption, a process where people experience great gain, there is no loss. That just isn't true.

To assume that all gain means only happiness is an illusion. To have such an illusion only serves to perpetuate the unfounded, imaginary fears that keep us from accepting reality.

"You Aren't Crazy, What You are Feeling is Normal"

When a survivor talks to us about the feelings that surround his or her loss, we often hear, "I don't know, I just feel crazy!" And too often, our response is, *"You aren't crazy! What you are feeling is quite normal."* That is a myth. The feelings that person is experiencing in the midst of the loss may very well be crazy to that person.

As the result of the death of a loved one, for instance, the bereaved person will experience any number of feelings. Some of these feelings will be new. Some of these feelings will be felt with more intensity than ever before. Certainly the bereaved will have feelings they aren't prepared to deal with. The feelings may seem to come at all the wrong times, as if there ever were a right time. The sad feelings come when the bereaved expects feelings of happiness; and contentment comes just when the bereaved can't imagine coping with another hour of pain. The widow feels a part of a couple still, but her husband no longer sits at the dinner table. The widower feels one with his wife still, but he climbs into bed alone at night. The divorcee feels the joy of her new-found freedom, and the sorrow of being alone, often at the same time. The man who recently lost his job imagines a world of opportunity at the same time he imagines his world collapsing all around him.

It is crazy! As one faces a loss and the task of working to re-identify who he or she is now, after that loss, one feels the fullness of the pain and happiness, the laughter and tears. He or she feels the craziness that is really a part of the grieving process at that time. It doesn't help us or others to deny that craziness. But we need to know the crazy feeling is a sign we are in the process of working to re-identify who we are now, as a result of our loss. If we accept our feelings for what they are, as a normal part of working through our grief, we can begin to see that this crazy time is not the time to be making major decisions in our lives. We are able to see some of the rocks, boulders and hazardous places in our everyday lives.

Accepting the craziness of grief is healthy because as we come to recognize this part of who we are, we can come to terms with the real work we will need to do to process our grief.

"Survivors Only Grieve for the Loss of the Dead."

Another terrible myth would suggest that for the most part, when a loved-one or a family member dies, all of our grief is for that family member. Or, in a divorce, when the kids move in with one parent, all they lose is the other parent. That is simply not true.

Richard J. Obershaw, MSW, LISCW

A family system —any relationship, for that matter— is much like a mobile. Have you ever seen a mobile hanging over a baby's crib? The mobile hangs there, nice and balanced with all those little giraffes and lions and tigers hanging at different levels, all balanced. What happens when you remove just one of those animals? The whole mobile goes cater-whompus. All of the animals get tangled up in each other and the mobile is a real mess.

It is the same thing when you look at relationships. When dad dies, you might hear people say to the kids, "Well, you still have Mom." That's only partly true. The kids may still have mom, but they will never have mom the way she used to be. When one parent dies the kids lose both of their parents. And, when parents divorce, the kids in the family lose both of their parents.

I heard it best from a six year old a few years ago. This little guy said to me, "You know, mommy isn't like mommy any more."

I asked the boy to tell me more and he continued, "Well, mommy used to pack my lunch everyday. She used to jam all kinds of things in there. I couldn't always eat it all. But now, since my dad moved away, some days, she forgets to even pack my lunch. She used to play with us a lot and read to us almost every night. But she doesn't hardly do that any more. She spends a lot of time at work now. I hardly ever see her." This child also lost his *mother* when his parents got a divorce. Dad moved away, so he lost his father, and mom is not the same person she used to be.

It is the same with loss due to death. It does not matter if the relationship is based in family or friendship. It does not matter if the bereaved is forty years old, or four years old. The reality is that when we lose someone close to us the loss is not limited to that one person. It affects us in our relationships with the others who have experienced that loss as well.

Problems Associated with These Myths

"But Dick, come on! Lil' ol' myths? What's the big deal?" I have been asked that often. And I do not need to answer, because, as I have already stated, *you* are already an expert on the subject of grief. You are already an expert on the myths of grief, and you know the added pain and suffering these myths can create. But let's review some of these problems in greater detail. Maybe, after we better understand the problems we create, we can begin to understand the importance of not perpetuating these myths.

The myth— *"Time Will Heal."*
The problems— Those who believe this myth will not do the *work* of grieving. They will seldom work to re-identify who they are following a loss. Also, and of major importance, the supportive network of family, friends, neighbors, and professionals will not put forth the work necessary to comfort the bereaved. This almost guarantees more isolation for the bereaved. If time does in fact heal, everyone can just stand back and wait for time to heal.

Richard J. Obershaw, MSW, LISCW

The myth— *"You'll Get Over It."*

The problems— If two, five or fifteen years after a loss, when the bereaved recall sentimental feelings about their loss, they may believe they carry around unresolved grief, or they are in some way unhealthy. Because the bereaved won't want others to know about their unhealthiness, they may quit communicating any of their normal and natural, everyday thoughts and feelings. That can indeed lead to a real unhealthiness! It will prevent them from telling others who they really are, and it may destroy or inhibit further interpersonal, intimate relationships.

A major loss in our life will affect us forever. We are, after all, made up of every experience we have ever survived. If someone tells you he is a survivor of WWII, you get to know a little bit more about that person. If someone tells you she is the mother of 12 children, the wife of an alcoholic, or the sister of a man who committed suicide, you get to know that person better. Our lives are changed forever by the experiences we survive. And often that change is for the better. It is a part of what makes us who we are today.

The myth— *"This is Just a Stage You are Going Through."*

The problems— Those who believe this myth feel that grief happens to them and they have no control over, or power in, the situation. This myth encourages feelings of helplessness. It may also lead to feelings of regression if you are angry immediately following a loss, and are then angry months later. Support people may not understand their role in the survivor's grief, and once again, expect the bereaved to pass through stages that just happen. And so, they may never get involved in comforting the bereaved.

The myth— *"True Believers Don't Cry."*
The problems— If the bereaved feel they have been faithful and devout to their God but are crying after a loss, and someone voices this myth to them, the bereaved may feel like they've lost their faith as well. The grief from multiple losses is more difficult to work through than that from a single loss.

Also, the bereaved may withdraw from the religious community and deny themselves the social and spiritual support so desperately needed at the time of loss.

The myth— *"Anticipated Grief is Easier to Handle."*
The problems— Believing this myth can cause the bereaved to think that they must be abnormal or emotionally unhealthy because they continue to feel sadness and pain long after they should be over their grief. When this occurs, the bereaved feel more crazy. Again, the network of supportive family and friends is less effective because they believe the bereaved should be all grieved out by now. If people believe this myth, they often do not realize the effect that grief will have on their work, their relationships, their concentration — all aspects of their lives— months or years after the recognized loss.

The myths—*"All Death Means Loss,"*
and *"All Gain Means Happiness."*

The problems—   If you do not understand the realities all loss means some gain and all gain means some loss, you may not accept all of the feelings that come with a change in your life. You may feel unhealthy when positive or happy feelings enter your life following a loss. Also, you may feel unhealthy when negative or sad feelings come after a major gain in your life.

The myth—   *"You Aren't Crazy, What You are Feeling is Normal"*
The problems—   When the bereaved feel lost and confused after a loss, they aren't feeling normal. To the bereaved, the grief that comes with a loss may feel quite crazy. When others try to assure them that these feelings are normal, the bereaved will not believe it. Consequently, they may avoid sharing the pain and suffering they feel because they don't want other to know how crazy they feel. This can lead the bereaved to withdraw to the point where no grief work is accomplished.

The myth—   *"Survivors Only Grieve for the Loss of the Dead."*
The problems—   If the bereaved only recognizes the major loss and not all of the assorted losses that accompany every major loss, they may not realize that the pain and suffering that could come weeks or months later is quite natural. Once again, the bereaved may feel they are not getting over their grief as they should.

        Also, if family and friends who work to comfort the bereaved do not recognize the losses that might accompany a major loss, the bereaved can be left feeling alone and completely misunderstood. Remember, if a child loses a father to death, that child also loses the person his mother used to be. The fullness of a loss often embodies more than just what we imagine to be the major loss. If we, grievers and supporters alike, diligently work to remind others about these myths, we can reduce our own needless suffering, protect others from the same, and get on with the task of working through grief.

The first thing we need to do to help eradicate these myths is not mouth them ourselves. Do not say these myths yourself, and when you hear them, correct the people who said them. Understand that when we suggest untruths about grief, we prolong the grieving process and cause more pain and suffering for the bereaved.

chapter six

Some Talk About Funerals

History of Funerals. Brief Group Reality Therapy. Professional Involvement. Committal Rites.

At some point in our lives, we will experience the loss of a loved one due to death, and for today, most of us just don't want to give that reality much thought. Hopefully, having read this book, you will have a better understanding of the work you can do to process grief in a healthy fashion, and consequently, have less fear of death and grief.

Likewise, at some point in our lives, we may find ourselves involved in planning a funeral for a family member or dear friend. And chances are, when that day does come, we will find ourselves unprepared for the work that will go into the very important ritual of the funeral. I hope that what I can share with you about the topic of funerals will prompt you to think about the valuable ceremony and ritual that funerals provide for the survivors of the death of a loved one.

History of Funerals

There are many people in the United States who believe that the only reason we have funerals is because funeral directors need them. There is no denying that caring for the dead has become a major business. But throughout the history of humankind, funerals have always been a major part of life. One need only to examine the famous burial tombs of rulers and pharaohs to realize that funerals have always been, and will always be, a vital part of humankind's dealing with life. To the best of my knowledge, there are no societies, peoples, tribes, groups or any other segment of society, that do not, in some fashion or form, memorialize, spiritualize, or finalize life following a death in their society.

Some of us witnessed funerals with less than five people in attendance, and most of us have been witness to funerals where millions were in attendance through the miracle of television. All of us, at some time, have either been at a funeral or can expect to attend one in the future. Some of us have the false impression that all funerals have to be religious in nature. Many funerals are political in nature. Some funerals are extremely hostile, while others may be a time for quiet meditation, for social reconstruction, or a time where survivors reflect on their own mortality. There are no recipes for the perfect funeral. All funerals should be specifically designed to meet the unique needs of the survivors.

Oftentimes, I believe that people have the mistaken idea that the funeral is for the deceased. It is important to know that the funeral has always been, and will always be, for the living. All the sociological, psychological, and spiritual needs that a funeral addresses are designed to meet the needs of the living. All of the needs of the one who has died have been met, and now, the funeral serves to meet the needs of those who have survived the death. Of course, there may be prayers for the dead; there may be offerings for the dead. But even these are made for the living. We must keep that in mind as we plan funerals. The funeral is a rite for the dead, and the funeral is a right of the survivors as well.

The rite of the funeral is a ceremony of incorporation for the dead. It is a process whereby the survivors move the deceased from the world of the living to the world of the dead. It is the survivor's right to acknowledge the death, to use the process to meet their psychological, spiritual, and sociological needs. And, it's interesting to note that the funeral is an affair where no one is formally invited, but all are expected to attend.

I believe that the funeral could be labeled as *Brief Grief Group Reality Therapy*. As a psychotherapist, I often hear people talk about the values of brief therapy, grief therapy, group therapy, the very important role of emotive therapy, and reality therapy. When the funeral is designed to meet the needs of the living, it can go a long way towards accomplishing what each of these treatments do on an individual basis.

Let us take a closer look at the components of *Brief Grief Group Reality Therapy*—

Brief Therapy

In our society, the funeral ritual and ceremony is usually quite brief. It begins with the making of funeral arrangements and generally concludes with the committal at a cemetery or the gathering of family and friends following the committal. This brief period may last only two or three days. And often that is not enough time for survivors to begin the healing process that must take place after a loss due to death.

In the past, the briefness or urgency of the funeral was based on the fact that society needed to rid itself of the dead body before it became a health hazard to the living. Today, with the modern sciences of embalming and preservation techniques, there is really no need to hurry this important ceremony. There is little need to make instant funeral arrangements. The deceased will be dead for a very long time, but the needs of the survivors will prevail.

Each of us can imagine that the grief of the survivors won't end after two or three days. As you read earlier, the work of grief can take place over a period of months or even years. The brief nature of the funeral marks the beginning of the work that each survivor will experience as they process their grief.

Grief Therapy

Grief therapy is the job of assisting others as they work to re-identify themselves following a significant loss. The funeral is an important part of this task. Immediately following a death, the survivors become survivors. They are responsible for making decisions that will affect their grief for the rest of their lives. The funeral they arrange or plan should be designed to meet the needs of all who survive the death.

After a death, we see people with tremendous amounts of grief, and we see people with very small amounts of grief. Still, we know that the funeral should be planned to meet the needs of all survivors. The funeral is a time where people come to recognize the reality of death and begin to deal with their suffering and pain surrounding their loss. To the survivors, funerals should be seen as a selfish act. As a survivor, it is our grief, our pain, and, it is our need to reorganize our selves. The funeral should be designed for those who attend. As I've suggested, grief is a very personal and individual job of re-identifying who we are after a loss. So, the funeral should also be as personal and individual as the needs of the survivors.

Group Therapy

The funeral is certainly group therapy. In many of the groups I have facilitated as a psychotherapist, I have found that it is important to deal with the reality of the group, the mixture of the group, the goals of the group, and the interactions of individual members within the group. In order to be successful, group therapy must address each of these. It is the same with a funeral.

After a death, numerous groups are affected. Sometimes, we make the mistake of thinking that there is only a family group: mother, father, sister, brother, grandchildren, parents. In reality, there are many groups that must be considered. There are friendship groups, working groups, religious groups, entertainment or social groups, political groups, and possibly, many other groups, all affected by the death. All of these groups have needs that must be met, and all should be informed of the death so each group can make plans to meet their common or individual needs.

There are groups within these groups. For example, there are groups of children, elderly and adults within a family group. In a religious group, there may be a group that encompasses an entire congregation, as well as a group of choir members or elders. As you can imagine, numerous groups will have numerous needs following a death. The funeral can be, and should be, designed to meet all of those needs. Sometimes, when planning a funeral, survivors err when they fail to remember the various groups that the deceased was a part of, and in doing so, may fall far short of meeting the very important needs of the survivors of the death.

Reality Therapy

Reality therapy is a type of treatment that has been in use for some time. It is a method that encourages patients to deal head-on with the reality of their particular situation in life. The funeral, when designed properly, is an excellent tool of reality therapy. With the dead body present at the funeral, the death is very real. It's hard to deny the reality of a death when you are at the funeral home during visitation and people are constantly talking about the deceased. "With this constant repetitive reminder of the death, the reality of the loss begins to slowly, but surely, sink into one's conscious awareness, and survivors can come to know that the person is really DEAD dead.

The very brief period of the funeral can gently bring survivors to the full reality of their significant loss. From the time of calling a funeral director, to completing funeral arrangements, to visiting with others at the funeral home, to confronting the dead human body, to marching down an aisle and recognizing the ritual or ceremony associated with the death, to going in procession to the place of final disposition of the dead human remains, to driving out of the cemetery; each of these serves to make the reality of the death that much more real. Without accepting that full reality, the bereaved find little desire to continue with their grief work.

The Parts of a Funeral

Obituary

The obituary —often called the death notice— is written in a newspaper or delivered over a local radio station. It simply reports that someone in the community has died, and may briefly list some of the survivors of the death. There is recognition of the value of obituaries. But, when you think about it, they serve a very important purpose to the survivors. The obituary serves as a very conspicuous S.O.S. —a plea for help, on the part of the survivors.

Let's take a closer look at the specific parts of the obituary. First, we have the name of the person who died; commonly called the "deceased." Immediately below that, we have the names of the family members who have survived the death. Following that, the obituary says, in essence, "We the survivors, who have lost big, need your handshakes, hugs, kisses, and comfort. Thus, we will be at such-and-such place at such-and-such time..."

This blatant call for help should remind us to always read obituaries, to always look for the survivors of death who will be asking us to be there when they need help and comfort in their time of pain and suffering. The obituary allows the survivors to issue a cry for help.

Richard J. Obershaw, MSW, LISCW

Funeral Arrangements

Making funeral arrangements is a very important task usually done by immediate family members. This task is important, in that it helps survivors come to terms with the reality of the death. It gives final closure to the life that has been lived, and helps in the very important task —that of redefining the family when one of its members is dead. As family members make funeral arrangements, the family restructures and redefines itself with the deceased family member no longer a part of the family group. Decisions must be made, people must be notified, expenses must be considered and plans for the new family group are often begun during the planning of a funeral.

If the deceased was the leader of the family, often these funeral arrangements are the first major decisions made by some other family member; and they will be difficult decisions. Often, the family will shift and maneuver and manipulate each other in the absense of the family leader who has died. Sometimes, families assemble together and take polls —in an indirect way— to determine who will become the new family leader. Some families find issues to fight over in order to make new leadership known. I've seen families fight over the color of the casket, the music that will be played, and the amount of money that will be spent. Although this seems to be traumatic and oftentimes, as reported by family members, feels to be irreverent, its a very good beginning to the restructuring that will go on between family members. So, the new family begins to reorganize as they make funeral arrangements.

Register Book

Those of you who have attended a funeral probably noticed the register book that was placed just outside or inside the door of the visitation room. It is an expected custom for those in attendance to sign their names in this book. Have you ever given any real thought to what the register book is doing there, or what purpose it serves?

The funeral is an occasion where no one is invited, but everyone is expected to attend. The register book suggests that you sign in so that the survivors, at a later date, can see if the comforters met their obligation. Since the funeral is a busy time when survivors are more occupied with re-identifying themselves than with who came or who didn't come to the funeral, the register book provides proof of one's attendance. I have known many survivors who couldn't remember the hundreds of people who came and helped them meet their needs at their time of loss, but cannot forget the one or two who failed to live up to their responsibility of attending the funeral.

Viewing the Body

We have all heard people say, *"I'm not going to view the dead body. I want to remember him or her as he or she was."*

This statement concerns me, as a therapist and as a human being. I know how important it is to have memories of others as they were when they lived. I am also cognizant of the fact that one has to remember the deceased for who they are now. When people die, they are no longer who they were. The reality is, they are now dead.

217

Richard J. Obershaw, MSW, LISCW

Viewing the dead body brings many interesting psychological and sociological ramifications with it. I have seen people yell at the deceased. I have seen others slap, kiss, or demand a response from the deceased. Of course, the dead cannot respond. This lack of response tells the survivors about the reality of death. When they see a dead body, they know that person is really DEAD dead.

When a body is placed in a open casket, it also serves as a focal point where the bereaved can gather to get support. The dead body can also help them initiate or even ignite their expressions of grief.

Viewing the dead body also assists the survivors as they bring closure to the relationship they had with the person when he or she was alive. This closure may come in the form of prayer. It may come in the form of messages given to the deceased that were never given while that person was alive. It may come in a pat or a kiss, as if to say, *"this is the end."* Viewing the body also tells the survivors they no longer need to ask the question, "Where is this person now, in my life?" The reality is before them.

There are some who would argue that viewing a body in a casket is unnatural because the body is clothed and may have some cosmetics applied. Some people suggest that such cosmetics or clothing is actually a denial of the reality of death. But when you think about it, almost all bodies in life have some form of cosmetic applied. If you men reading this are skeptical, let me remind you that you probably have some form of deodorant on your body now. This

218

may be a denial of life, but for the most part, it makes oneself more acceptable to others. This is what positioning and cosmeticizing a dead human's remains does —it makes the dead body more acceptable to those still living. The body that is clean and positioned in a way that suggests no pain or suffering is more acceptable to others. Others may find it easier to be around, to identify with, to touch, and to integrate the true reality of the death. Consider a closed casket lid as the thickest layer of cosmetic you can use when it comes to viewing the reality of death.

Also, being able to see the dead body brings an end to the search that goes on for many survivors following a death. All the soldiers listed as Missing In Action, remind us how important finding the dead and accepting their death truly is. By seeing the body and touching the body, our search can come to an end.

Organization/Direction

When one loses, one has a tendency to feel very disorganized. The funeral can help survivors with that disorganization. A funeral is a very organized, purposeful, group-centered, time-limited response to a major loss, according to Dr. Paul Irion. One of the reasons we call a funeral director a director is because he or she gives direction at a time when one is very disorganized and without direction. This direction, if given in a professional sense, aids the survivors as they work to process the pain of their grief in a very purposeful way.

Richard J. Obershaw, MSW, LISCW

The funeral is often organized from a religious, or spiritual standpoint. Almost all religions have some plan or procedure, ritual or ceremony that is faithfully followed after a death. This tells the bereaved that there is organization all around them at a time when they feel so terribly disorganized. Around the funeral, friends, neighbors, co-workers, and others provide organized responses to the bereaved in their hour of need. I can't begin to tell you how many widows I have worked with who reported that in their deepest hour of sorrow and disorganization, they were so grateful to have been able to make organized decisions with the help of professionals and other family members. This gave them the knowledge that they could make organized decisions in the future.

Professional Involvement

Throughout the process of funeral planning, arranging, directing and officiating, professionals are constantly involved with the survivors who represent the deceased. In the past, these professionals have always been the clergy and funeral directors. Today, this community of professionals has grown to include nurses and physicians, hospital chaplains, social workers and volunteers who work in the area of oncology, long-term care, and hospice.

During the funeral, many of these people have contact with the survivors and can see where the survivors are in the process of working through their grief. By being involved in the funeral, and by having professionals around to support them, survivors can avoid some of the pit falls that may lead to serious problems in the future. These professionals can assist survivors as they process grief, they can help family members as they work together in the new family group, and they can provide valuable support to the bereaved.

Post-funeral follow-up by funeral directors, clergy, hospice volunteers and social workers can also be very valuable to survivors. In many cases, people stop ritualizing immediately following the funeral, and often, healing stops altogether. The professionals involved may create other rituals and ceremonies to assist the survivors in the vacant weeks and months that often follow the funeral.

The Cortege

The cortege, or processional, as it is often called, is also a valuable part of the funeral service. It is here that the body is moved from the world of the living to the world of the dead. The processional often moves from a funeral home to a place of worship, then on to the cemetery. This procession shows the community of the living that a death has occurred and that there are a number of people affected by this death. It also reports to the community that death is still a constant reality of life. Without the funeral procession, many people would not be reminded of the reality of death in our society today.

The procession is as important to the survivors as it is to the larger community. Many times, survivors feel that life for them has ended because of the tragedy and pain of their loss. As the procession moves slowly through the streets, communities, and neighborhoods on the way to the cemetery, survivors are reminded that the world continues on around them, even though they feel it should end. So in the throes of their grief, survivors are reminded that life continues on.

The processional is also beneficial from a safety standpoint. The procession allows a very orderly, directed, and organized flow of the bereaved from the place of service to the place of final disposition. If one leaves the bereaved family members and friends to find their own way in this, their deepest hour of sorrow, it is quite evident that many hazardous and dangerous circumstances could occur. The processional, in its organized and safety-conscious manner, moves those who are grieving safely to their destination. Grief is often a period of preoccupation, disorganization, and confused thinking for the bereaved. And that is not a good time to place these individuals behind the wheel of an automobile without direction and guidance.

Committal Rites

When the survivors have completed the initial tasks of grieving-in part, by confronting the reality of the death the dead body must be disposed of The body can be cremated, donated to a school of medical science, or buried in a cemetery. At the final place of disposition, the rites of committal are usually completed. This committal allows for family members to come to the full realization that they are giving up or losing that body and the ability to view that body. This can help survivors come to grips with the finality and reality of the death. It also brings together a group of people who can be of some support to the survivors.

Donation or cremation of the body does not preclude a committal rite or ceremony. These religious or humanistic services can be carried out at the place of cremation or donation. If you remember that searching is a major part of the grieving process, you can understand that this committal ceremony brings family and friends together at the place of committal. This will assist survivors in the future because they will know exactly where to go when they feel a need to search.

Also, the future is made more secure for survivors by marking this place of final disposition. With a tombstone, headstone, or even a small marker, the survivors will have this place marked forever.

Post-Funeral Gathering

Following the rites of final disposition or committal, the survivors often reassemble in an orderly fashion, either at the church or synagogue, a family member's home, or another meeting place. During this time, family members share food and drink, and reminisce about the deceased. Sometimes, survivors get upset because people talk about the humorous experiences they recall with the deceased. Often, these conversations are very light-hearted and not at all serious. I believe that this merry-making may be one of the more significant signs that the funeral has done its job. When the grief following the initial pain of loss has been processed in a healthy fashion, survivors are often able to come together to share the more joyous occasion of life. Old relationships are re-examined, old memories are re-told, and reorganization is begun.

Richard J. Obershaw, MSW, LISCW

Cost

Funerals can cost anywhere from a few hundred dollars to several thousands of dollars. Decisions about cost should be based on the family's wishes and desires. A funeral that costs several thousand dollars, but does not include any arrangement by family members —no viewing of the body, no final disposition rites or cortege, and no final family gathering— would probably be a major waste of money. On the other hand, a funeral that may be much less expensive, but includes all of the above, could be of tremendous value.

Just as all families have different values and different standards of living, so too does a funeral have different requirements to different people, according to their own standards. For some people, a very inexpensive casket states their values, as well as their perception of their own needs. To others, a very expensive casket may state their perception of how the deceased lived, as well as reflect their standard of living.

Funerals, their simplicity or their elaborateness, are often a true reflection of the deceased's lifestyle, as well as the lifestyle of the survivors. Seldom, if ever, do people living in poverty have extremely expensive funerals. And seldom, if ever, do people who are very rich have very inexpensive funerals. The image of a funeral director gouging poor widows out of their money for elaborate funeral expenses is just not reality. Every funeral director I have ever known is aware that he or she cannot repossess the merchandise following a burial. It does not make sense for them to encourage survivors to spend money they do not have for such services.

I would imagine that an average cost of a funeral today would run about $3,000.00. If that funeral is attended by 150 people, that would bring the average cost per person to $20. If the funeral is designed to meet the needs of all survivors, you can see how inexpensive —or cost-effective, per person— that period of brief grief group reality therapy really is. It's much cheaper, in the long run, to make the most of this valuable tool, when you compare that cost to seeing a professional grief therapist at $90 per hour. If, on the other hand, the needs of the survivors are not met by the funeral, it doesn't matter how much money is spent; it will have been a waste of money.

As a psychotherapist and grief counselor, I have worked for over 20 years in the area of grief and bereavement counseling. I have seen many people make major blunders when they try to short-circuit the rite, and right, of the funeral service. Whenever that happens, the blunders almost always come back to haunt the survivors. And in the long run, it increases the survivor's chances of having unresolved grief and the need to seek professional counseling. I encourage you to try to understand the dynamics of the funeral; to truly use the funeral for all that it can provide in the resolution of grief following a death.

I hope you understand the important role a funeral plays for the survivors of death. And, I ask you to consider the fact that the needs of the survivors are constantly changing. If a funeral is planned ahead, even planned ahead by someone anticipating their own death, all too often the needs of the survivors are completely ignored. I don't mean to suggest that families shouldn't put money aside to cover the expenses of a funeral; that is only prudent. But, to plan a funeral in anticipation of a death doesn't take into account the needs of the survivors. After all, the funeral isn't for the deceased. They will have no needs after they are dead; they will not care about the color of their caskets or the selection of music played during visitation.

The funeral is for the *survivors of a death.* It should make your eyes wet —and cleanse them to better see the future.

When the funeral is used in a healthy manner, survivors can be cleansed as they begin that long, arduous process of redefining who they are now, after their loss. The funeral should provide a safe environment for all survivors, family members, groups, and individuals. All who attend should be able to express all of their pain and sorrow, as well as their hope and joy.

When survivors realize that the funeral has helped them learn that they can and will continue to live, it will have been a major factor in helping them deal with their pain and sorrow. The funeral is one ritual and ceremony that must be planned and conducted with a great deal of thought and care for the survivors...

The End,
The Beginning

The preceding pages have been filled with words; black dots of ink on paper. Your eyes have read these words, and your brain has interpreted them according to your life experiences. Some of the same words that brought you feelings of sadness brought other readers in touch with feelings of joy or hope. As you work to re-identify yourself following a loss, you too may be surprised that the stimuli that caused you to feel pain yesterday may help you to feel renewed hope tomorrow.

Perhaps you should put this book down for now and mark your calendar for 90 days from today. On that day, go back and re-read some of these same black dots of ink on paper and see how far you've come in reidentifying yourself after your loss.

After all, it is your life.

And you are a survivor.

bibliography

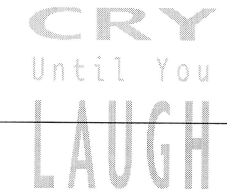

Holmes and Machoeski,
"The Social Readjustment Scale,"
JOURNAL OF PSYCHOSOMATIC RESEARCH
[April, 1967, *pages 213-218*]

Irion, Paul.,
The Funeral: Vestige or Value?
[Abingdon Press, Nashville, 1966]

Kübler-Ross, Elisabeth, M.D.,
On Death and Dying
[MacMillan, New York, 1969 (*1974 ed.*)]

Kusner, Herold,
When Bad Things Happen to Good People
[Schocken Books, New York, 1981]

Parks, Collin,
Bereavement: Studies of Grief in Adult Life
[International Universities Press, New York, 1973]

Worden, James,
Grief Counseling and Grief Therapy,
[Springer Publishing Co., New York, 1982]

about the author

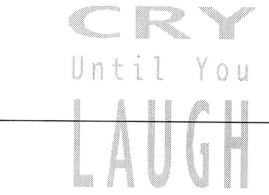

RICHARD J. OBERSHAW, MSW, LICSW, is highly qualified to address the topics of Grief and Death in our society today. He holds degrees in Psychology, Mortuary Science, and Social Work. He presently serves as founder and director of The Grief Center and Burnsville Counseling Clinic in Burnsville, Minnesota, where he has a full-time private psychotherapy practice and serves as clinic administrator. A popular speaker, Mr. Obershaw travels and lectures across the United States and Canada to professional, corporate, and lay groups on the topics of death, grief, stress, personality issues, and other related topics. He lives in Burnsville, Minnesota.

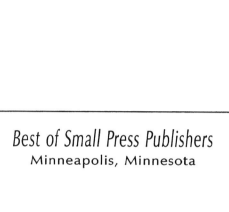

Best of Small Press Publishers
Minneapolis, Minnesota